**Model Systems in
Biological Psychiatry**

**Model Systems in
Biological Psychiatry**

Edited by
David J. Ingle and
Harvey M. Shein

The MIT Press
Cambridge, Massachusetts,
and London, England

This book was set in CRT Times Roman,
printed on Fernwood Black and White Smooth,
and bound in Columbia Millbank Vellum MBV 4750,
by The Colonial Press, Inc.,
in the United States of America.

Library of Congress Cataloging in Publication Data
Main entry under title:

Model systems in biological psychiatry.

"Symposium organized by Drs. Ingle and Shein and published in this volume."
Includes index.
1. Mental illness—Physiological aspects—Congresses. 2. Comparative
psychiatry—Congresses. 3. Neurobiology—Congresses. 4. Biological models—Congresses.
I. Ingle, David, ed. II. Shein, Harvey M., ed. [DNLM: 1. Disease models, Animal. 2.
Mental disorders. 3. Models, Biological. WM100 I51m]
RC455.4.B5M62   616.8′9′00184   74-32500
ISBN 0-262-09015-5

Contents

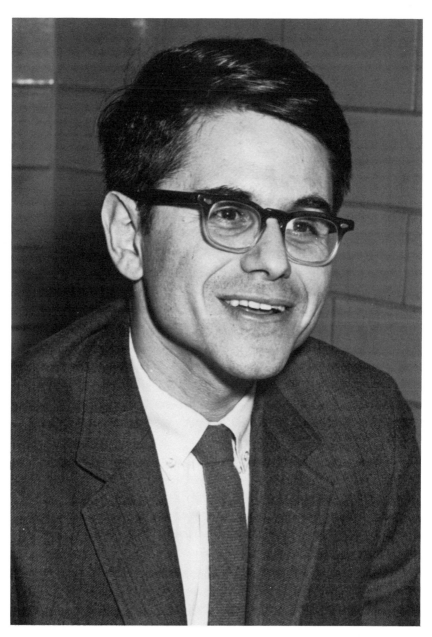

Harvey M. Shein
1933–1974

Dedication

Harvey M. Shein died suddenly on July 18, 1974, in Boston. His death came as a shock to his colleagues, including some of the participants in the present symposium with whom he had had many close interactions. Because of our friendship, and because we regard Harvey as exemplifying the interdisciplinary spirit that has motivated this book, we would like to dedicate it to his memory. Toward that end we have asked Professor Alfred Pope, who closely followed Harvey Shein's research at McLean Hospital, to compose the following summary of his career.

David Ingle

The Work of Harvey M. Shein

With the death of Harvey Shein the worlds of neuroscience and psychiatry have lost an extraordinarily gifted and accomplished physician-scientist, whose intellect and industry led him to pursue simultaneous careers in cell biology and psychiatry, either one of which would have qualified him for a significant place in the annals of these disciplines. Together they resulted in a unique, though all too brief, professional life, full of notable achievements and of future promise.

Dr. Shein's development as a scientist had its roots in his devotion, while an undergraduate at Cornell, to philosophy, and particularly to the thought of Ludwig Wittgenstein. As a student at Harvard Medical School he carried out special studies under the guidance of Professor John F. Enders, and he continued this training during a postgraduate year as a research fellow. In the course of this work he was the first to achieve transformation of human kidney cells cultured in vitro by the action of an oncogenic virus.

He managed to continue this productive association while an intern in medicine at Beth Israel Hospital and during the first years of his residency in psychiatry at McLean Hospital. Then, during 1964 and

1965, he established his own unit for tissue culture and virology in the McLean Hospital Biological Research Laboratory. Here he embarked on an extensive series of investigations on the pathobiology, biochemistry, and pharmacology of brain cellular species cultures in vitro, while at the same time completing his education in psychiatry and psychoanalysis and advancing in both clinical and academic hierarchies to positions of major responsibility in patient care, research, and education. His rapid progress from resident psychiatrist to major academic and service roles at McLean and Harvard Medical School, coupled with his maturation and productivity as a neuroscientist, constitute a remarkable record of professional achievement.

Dr. Shein began his work at McLean with a series of studies on the biology and pathology of human and animal astroglia in vitro, and on the neoplastic transformations induced in them by oncogenic viruses. His isolation of dispersed cell lines of fetal astrocytes and his successful viral induction of experimental gliomas in vitro were widely recognized as virtuoso accomplishments in neurological cell biology. The cultured cell lines thus established were extensively studied by Dr. Shein in collaboration with colleagues in the McLean laboratories and elsewhere and have yielded important information on the biochemistry and quantitative histochemistry of normal and neoplastic neuroglia. At the same time his ingenious utilization of organ cultures of the pineal gland as a particularly suitable model system for studies on biogenic-amine metabolism resulted in a second in vitro paradigm for analysis of the metabolic pathways important in neurobiology. This model was extensively exploited, particularly in collaboration with Julius Axelrod and Richard Wurtman and their associates, for analysis of the steps in neurotransmitter synthesis and of the metabolic loci of action of psychopharmacological agents.

Many other investigations might also be cited to indicate the broad impact of Dr. Shein's studies on the cellular physiology and pathology of the nervous system. His was a truly pioneering role at the advancing frontiers between cell biology and both neuropathology and psycho-pharmacology. It is remarkable that he developed conceptual capabilities for creative leadership in the latter fields as well as in those with which he is especially identified.

Dr. Shein's intellectual endeavors were by no means limited to his laboratory investigations, but included as well valuable contributions to the literature of clinical psychiatry. His extensive list of publications also includes thoughtful reviews on tissue culture of the nervous system and on the oncogenic and other long-term effects of chronic viral infections of the brain. In its entirety this list speaks for itself regarding Dr. Shein's effectiveness and versatility as a psychiatrist and neuroscientist.

The symposium organized by Drs. Ingle and Shein and published in this volume is itself a clear reflection of Harvey Shein's intense interest in applying neurobiology to illnesses of the human mind. It is, therefore, in every way fitting and proper that it be dedicated to the memory of this remarkable physician and biologist.

Alfred Pope
McLean Hospital

1
Introduction

David J. Ingle and Harvey M. Shein

This is a book about model systems and how they are used by experimentalists who wish to isolate biological phenomena relating to both normal mental functioning and the pathophysiology of mental disorders. The book does not attempt to review or justify theoretical models of the mind, of the brain, or of specific diseases. The contributors have each sought an appropriate experimental vehicle—a specific laboratory preparation—for explorations that may help both to define relevant biological correlates of behavior and to assist in the conceptual integration of the many factors leading to mental illness.

In most other areas of medical research the use of model systems is a well-worn habit and scarcely needs introduction or justification. The student of cancer, for example, has genetically homogeneous rodent or avian strains that reliably develop certain types of cancer, or respond to carcinogens in a well-known manner, or spontaneously emit oncogenic viruses. It is less clear to the psychiatrist that he can identify in simpler model systems those derangements that appear uniquely "human." It is still all too easy in psychiatry to utilize in a constraining manner the conventional wisdom that "the proper study of mankind is man" and to give insufficient attention to the present and potential contributions of animal psychologists, physiologists, pharmacologists, and molecular biologists.

Many of the contributors to the workshop of which this book is a record are psychiatrists or psychologists who desire to avoid using exclusively verbal formulas as explanatory constructs; they therefore work in addition as laboratory scientists in order to gain a firmer understanding of the biological bases of the psychopathological phenomena that interest them. More often than not the scientist-psychiatrist will select a topic that is viewed as a fundamental problem in neurobiology. He may thus, for example, choose to explore the biological correlates of schizophrenia by studying the interactions of psychoactive drugs with brain monoamine neurotransmitter systems that have been observed to be altered by these drugs in patients. Similarly he may choose to approach aggression by examining functional correlates of the various hypothalamofugal pathways observed to be related to aggressive behaviors. He may even choose to seek out biological correlates of aberrant memory by studying the macromolecular basis of synaptic plasticity.

The present workshop grew out of the realization that there were several research psychiatrists in and near the Boston area who were trying to develop clearer correlations between clinical and laboratory problems by working upon simpler systems that "model" various interesting clinical issues. The workshop brought some of these scientist-clinicians together with biologically oriented behaviorists with the aim of making more explicit the advantages of working with model systems in biological psychiatry.

Work in biological psychiatry has recently tended to cluster within a few areas of increasing popularity: (1) mechanisms of drug action in the brain; (2) effects of biochemical and surgical manipulations of the brain on motivational components of animal behavior; (3) effects of early environment upon animal behavior and brain function; (4) ethological studies of mother-offspring relations and social structures; (5) genetics of animal and human behavior; and (6) neurophysiological studies of phenomena related to attention, habituation, and learning. Much of this work has been heuristically motivated by two widely accepted assumptions: (1) animal brains and animal behavior closely model phenomena of basic importance in human development and in the expression of human psychopathology; and (2) in order to develop in systematic fashion progressively more useful concepts concerning the biological bases of psychopathology it is essential to utilize simpler animal and in vitro models to pull apart and analyze in detail the relevant isolable neural circuits and biochemical events.

Given this attitude and the variety of new laboratory methods available to study the brain and to dissect behavior, how does one go about choosing a "model system"? The specific answer must be derived from the particular "clinical" phenomenon to be explained—as each of the following chapters will illustrate—but there are some ground rules that seem to apply quite broadly. Simplicity and technical convenience are the fundamental considerations, although the simplified model must always retain at least a few essential characteristics of the system being modeled (e.g., man). Thus, for most biological studies of biochemical or neural phenomena, phylogenetically lower species are generally preferred. However, if one ventures too far from the mammalian group, the basic design of the brain changes radically and the behavioral and biological elements are more difficult to homologize with man.

In general, the model systems of clinically oriented researchers reflect a compromise between the advantages of experimental simplicity and those of similarity (or homology) of model functions to functions manifest in human behavior. The conflicts inherent in such a compromise invite no general solution since there is a need for "models" for a wide variety of basic, as well as clinically relevant, research problems. At this still early stage of model-system construction in psychiatry, we hope that the inclusion in this volume of model systems illustrative of each of these contrasting categories will stimulate the imaginations of prospective researchers.

2
Animal Models of Schizophrenia

Steven Matthysse and Suzanne Haber

Abnormal behavior in animals can be provoked by a variety of pharmacological, environmental, and genetic interventions. If any of these abnormal states could be considered analogues to schizophrenia, they would provide models with both practical and theoretical value in screening new psychotherapeutic drugs and in suggesting neural pathways that might be disturbed in schizophrenia. The chief obstacle to the use of these models lies in the difficulty of establishing their relevance to human psychopathology. One might, of course, sidestep the question by giving abnormal animal behavior a noncommittal name and studying it as a phenomenon in its own right; but our interest in its physiology and pharmacology would be much greater if we had grounds to believe that this behavior is really analogous to some aspect of schizophrenia.

It is possible to establish some criteria that a model behavior should satisfy in order to be a useful analogy to schizophrenia for the purpose of testing antipsychotic drugs or formulating hypotheses about pathophysiology. These are necessary, rather than sufficient, conditions; as will become evident from the review of the literature which follows, however, they are not easy to satisfy.

1. *The aberrant animal behavior ought to be restored to normal, at least in part, by drugs which are known to be effective in the treatment of schizophrenia.* Furthermore among these drugs there are well-established potency ratios (Davis, 1974), and these relative potencies should also characterize their normalizing effects on the animal model (unless species differences in drug metabolism account for the discrepancies). For example, haloperidol is as much as fifty times as potent as chlorpromazine in milligram potency in man, and we should expect this ratio to

S. Matthysse, Psychiatric Research Laboratories, Massachusetts General Hospital, Boston, MA, 02114. S. Haber, Department of Psychiatry, Stanford University, Stanford, CA, 94305.

be maintained in the animal model unless a reason for the exception can be found.

2. *Drugs closely related in chemical structure to the antipsychotic phenothiazines and butyrophenones, but without efficacy in the treatment of psychosis, ought also to be without normalizing effect in the animal model.*

It is possible that the action of a tranquilizing drug on a pathological animal behavior is related to a side effect of this drug in man, rather than to its antipsychotic effect; for example, many tranquilizers are also sedatives and might normalize behavior merely by lowering the animal's level of arousal. Fortunately the characteristic side effects of tranquilizers are shared by drugs with closely related structures that do not have an antipsychotic effect, and these latter drugs can be used to test the side-effect hypothesis. The sedative effect of chlorpromazine, for example, is shared by promethazine, a nonantipsychotic phenothiazine. We should insist that promethazine *not* normalize the deviant animal behavior. This criterion is especially useful because, in the hundreds of drug trials that have been conducted since the introduction of the phenothiazines in 1955, a fairly clear dichotomy between antipsychotic and nonantipsychotic phenothiazines has emerged.

The nonantipsychotic phenothiazines mimic several important side-effect dimensions of tranquilizing drugs; among them are sedatives (e.g., promethazine), antihistaminics (e.g., trimeprazine), and anticholinergics (e.g., ethopropazine). Some induce the parkinsonian motor symptoms characteristic of antipsychotic drugs (e.g., thiethyl-perazine). The fact that their effects vary along several dimensions creates the possibility of controlling for these dimensions of tran-quilizing drug activity in designing animal experiments. If anti-psychotic drugs normalize a pathological animal behavior, and if the effect is not sedative, anticholinergic, antihistaminic, or extrapyramidal, there is reason to hope it is related to whatever property of the tranquilizers makes them antipsychotic.

This criterion, which we propose for evaluating the relevance of behavioral effects of tranquilizing drugs, has been applied before to their biochemical effects (Matthysse, 1973), and in that realm it is very stringent. Electron-donor capacity, inhibition of oxidative phosphorylation, and stabilization of membranes—biochemical effects that are well known to be characteristic of tranquilizing drugs—all fail to distinguish between the antipsychotic and nonantipsychotic phenothiazines. Acceleration of dopamine synthesis and utilization, however, does for the most part satisfy the criterion, with a few exceptions that remain unexplained (Matthysse, 1974).

3. *Tolerance (the tendency, after repeated doses of a drug, to require an increased dose to produce the same effect) should not develop to the behavior-normalizing effect of tranquilizers in the animal model since it does not develop to their antipsychotic action.* This is a powerful criterion because the sedative effects of tranquilizing drugs in man do show tolerance, unlike their antipsychotic actions, so that in this way the sedative and antipsychotic dimensions can be distinguished.

4. *The normalizing effects of tranquilizers on the abnormal animal behavior should not be blocked by the simultaneous administration of anticholinergic agents.* The rationale for this principle lies in the frequent clinical use of anticholinergics as an adjunct to phenothiazines or butyrophenones, in order to counteract the parkinsonian side effects of these drugs, with no apparent diminution of their antipsychotic activity. This principle, therefore, permits us to separate the antipsychotic and extrapyramidal dimensions of the tranquilizing drugs.

A certain amount of caution is necessary in applying this principle. A recent study (which, unfortunately, was not double-blind) did find a reduction of antipsychotic effects following the simultaneous administration of anticholinergics (Singh and Smith, 1973). Hostile, uncooperative behavior reappeared after anticholinergic administration, but disorders of perception did not. The criterion is more difficult to apply experimentally than the others since two drugs must be administered in appropriate time and dose relationships. Nevertheless, it may be a useful supplement to the other principles.

These criteria, which we propose to apply to animal models of schizophrenia, amount to a requirement of *isomorphism* in the mathematical sense. Each formal characteristic of one system is required to have an exact counterpart in another, although the objects contained in the two systems may not be alike. In our case the two systems are the clinical phenomena of schizophrenia and the animal behavior selected as a model; the formal characteristics that are required to be preserved in going from one system to the other are the responses to pharmacological intervention.

The value of the isomorphism criteria derives from the importance of homology in the evolution of the brain. In the course of the extensive development of the nervous system during mammalian evolution, the spatial locations of nuclear groups changed and the cytoarchitectonic structure became increasingly complex. The possibility of an animal model rests upon the fact that, despite this evolution, not everything changed. Structures homologous to many of the major nuclear groups of the human brain can be found in lower mammals: for example, structures similar with respect to patterns of interconnection, locations in the embryonic primordia, and (especially important for our purpose) the utilization of neurotransmitters. Schizophrenia must be associated with functional alterations in (yet unknown) neural structures or pathways, and if some behavior in a lower mammal is associated with the activity of the structures and pathways homologous to these, it ought to show pharmacological isomorphism.

We have undertaken a review of the literature on the effects of tranquilizing drugs in animals in order to find out whether any of the behavioral models so far investigated satisfy the isomorphism criteria. In many cases the decisive experiments have not been done; in others isomorphism can be excluded on the basis of existing experiments. None of the behaviors we have reviewed can be shown to satisfy the criteria fully. Our conclusions are summarized in Table 2.1. Each of these models will now be considered in more detail.

Table 2.1
The isomorphism criteria: a review of the literature

Behavior	Potency correlation	Absence of influence by nonantipsychotics	Absence of tolerance	Absence of anticholinergic blockade
Stereotypy	?	(−)	−	−
Arousal	−	−	−	(−)
Self-stimulation	+	?	?	−
Operant performance	−	−	?	?
Conditioned avoidance	+	?	?	(−)

Notation: +: experimental results appear to satisfy the criterion;
  −: experimental results appear not to satisfy the criterion;
  ?: no data or conflicting data;
  ( ): existing data, while suggestive, is inconclusive.

Stereotypy Induced by Amphetamine or Apomorphine

As Randrup (1974) has emphasized, stereotypy induced by amphetamine or apomorphine is, not a new behavior, but the repetitive and exaggerated performance of any one element of the animal's repertoire to the exclusion of others. The behavioral element that is repeated may differ from individual to individual, and from trial to trial for a given individual. Rats tend to sniff, lick, and gnaw. Monkeys, having a more complex repertoire, are less predictable, although once a stereotyped pattern emerges it will be performed repetitiously and compulsively. Stereotyped grooming and staring are particularly common. Humans also exhibit stereotyped behavior in response to psychotomimetic doses of amphetamines; the presence of this phenomenon in man has, naturally, greatly contributed to its importance as a model of schizophrenic psychoses. Ellinwood and coworkers (1973) describe examples of such amphetamine-induced stereotypes in man as "repetitious stringing of beads . . . lining up pebbles, rocks or other small objects . . . taking apart such objects as television sets, watches, radios, and phonographs. Subsequently, the parts may be analyzed, arranged, sorted, filed, and cataloged and, rarely, put back together."

It is true, in a general way, that antipsychotic drugs block amphetamine- and apomorphine-induced stereotyped behavior (Janssen et al., 1967). The unresolved questions concern the exactness of the correlation between clinical potency and stereotypy blockade. In this respect thioridazine and thiethylperazine are two drugs that pose dilemmas. Thioridazine is a well-recognized antipsychotic, generally regarded as equal in milligram potency to chlorpromazine (Davis, 1974). Some clinicians regard it as less effective with very disturbed patients, but the probable explanation is the dosage ceiling imposed by thioridazine's side effects. Thiethylperazine is a phenothiazine valued in clinical practice for its antiemetic effects, but not generally regarded as antipsychotic (although there is one report of its successful use in the treatment of schizophrenia, based on a nonblind study (Vencovsky, 1967)). Thioridazine has a stereotypy-blocking effect in rats much too low relative to its clinical potency, whereas the blocking effect of thiethylperazine is much too high (Janssen et al., 1967). Some results in the dog (Rotrosen et al., 1972) and pigeon (Gupta and Dhawan, 1965) are more in accord with the clinical effectiveness of thioridazine; thiethylperazine has, thus far, not been studied in animals other than the rat.

The relevance of amphetamine- or apomorphine-induced stereotyped behavior as an animal model of schizophrenia is called into question by the development of tolerance to the blocking effects of antipsychotic drugs. Tolerance might have been expected, because prolonged treatment of guinea pigs with chlorpromazine (Klawans and Rubovits, 1972) and of rats with haloperidol (Asper et al., 1973) decreases the dose of apomorphine or amphetamine required to induce stereotyped behavior. Some authors attribute the decrease in threshold to hypersensitivity of dopamine receptors analogous to acetylcholine-receptor hypersensitivity following neuromuscular denervation, but this mechanism is not proved. Tolerance has been shown to develop in three experimental systems (Møller Nielsen et al., 1974): blockade by haloperidol of amphetamine stereotypy in rats; by pimozide of apomorphine stereotypy in rats; and by fluphenazine of methylphenidate stereotypy in mice. The doses of neuroleptics used to induce tolerance in rats were high (10 mg/kg haloperidol and 2.5 mg/kg pimozide p.o.), but the dose of fluphenazine used in mice was somewhat closer to the clinical range (0.31 mg/kg p.o.).

Stereotypy also seems to violate the fourth criterion, resistance to blockade of neuroleptic drug effects by anticholinergics. Scopolamine significantly reduced the inhibiting effect of haloperidol on methylphenidate-induced gnawing in mice (both nontolerant and haloperidol-tolerant mice showed this antagonism) (Fjalland and Møller Nielsen, 1974). Similar results have been obtained by other experimenters (Morpurgo and Theobald, 1964; Arnfred and Randrup, 1968). The paradoxical effects of thioridazine and thiethylperazine, the development of tolerance, and the blockade of neuroleptic effects by anticholinergics, all suggest that this popular model, despite its intrinsic interest, has only limited relevance to schizophrenia. We will discuss later some modifications of the stereotypy model that might make it more applicable.

Catalepsy (a state of immobility in which abnormal postures can be maintained for an unnatural period of time) is sometimes regarded as the pharmacological converse of stereotypy, since many of the drugs that block stereotypy will produce catalepsy in high doses. Antagonism of neuroleptic-induced catalepsy by anticholinergics has been observed (Morpurgo, 1964). The literature on tolerance to induction of catalepsy is inconclusive. In one study the cataleptogenic effect of 1.5 mg/kg p.o. haloperidol in rats decreased by 50% after treatment for 21 days (Asper et al., 1973). In another investigation with the same drug and in the same species, tolerance did not develop after 10 mg/kg p.o. for 12 days (Møller Nielsen et al., 1974). Further experiments are needed to evaluate catalepsy from the point of view of the isomorphism criteria.

Some additional effects of apomorphine that are antagonized by neuroleptics include induction of emesis (Cook et al., 1958), provocation of aggression in confined animals (Senault, 1970), and lowering of body temperature when animals are kept in a cold environment (Barnett et al., 1972). If it is accepted that thiethylperazine, despite its potent antiemetic activity, is not antipsychotic, emesis does not seem to be a satisfactory model. The aggression and hypothermic effects also do not appear to satisfy the criteria (Cook et al., 1958; Barnett et al., 1972).

Arousal
Effects on activity level in animals would not be expected to provide a good model for the antipsychotic actions of the phenothiazines since it is well known that, clinically, sedative and antipsychotic effects can be separated. Experimental studies are in accord; for example, thioridazine is less effective than chlorpromazine in suppressing the activity level of several species (Shillito, 1967), tolerance develops to the suppression of activity level by chlorpromazine in rats (Boyd, 1960), and anticholinergic agents antagonize the locomotor-depressant effects of several phenothiazines (Morpurgo and Theobald, 1964).

An interesting variation on the study of arousal is self-administration of amphetamine by monkeys through an indwelling intravenous catheter. Under certain conditions chlorpromazine, despite its generally depressant effect on behavior, enhances the rate of self-administration of amphetamine, as if the animals were attempting to maintain a constant arousal level. It is interesting that tolerance did not develop after five days of chlorpromazine injections, but the comparative drug studies have not been done that would be needed to demonstrate that this effect is not merely a response to sedation (Wilson and Schuster, 1972).

A thoughtful interpretation of the role of arousal in schizophrenia underlies the work of Kornetsky and his colleagues, who have regarded arousal as an intervening variable in the capacity for sustained attention as measured by the continuous performance test (CPT). They have concluded that an intermediate level of arousal is optimal for attention. Thus errors of omission in the CPT are increased by chlorpromazine in rats, monkeys, and man (Kornetsky and Bain, 1965; Mirsky and Bloch, 1967; Latz and Kornetsky, 1965). Conversely, if a state of hyperarousal is induced by stimulation of the mesencephalic reticular formation in rats, omission errors on the CPT increase, and a dose of chlorpromazine that would under normal conditions impair performance now improves it. These observations led Kornetsky's group to surmise that schizophrenics are in a chronic state of hyperarousal which impairs their attention and hence their cognitive processes, and that this state is alleviated by chlorpromazine (Kornetsky and Eliasson, 1969).

The obvious question concerning the actions of chlorpromazine on CPT performance is whether or not they are sedative effects. It is noteworthy that barbiturates do not have a marked effect on omission errors (Kornetsky and Bain, 1965; Mirsky and Bloch, 1967; Latz and Kornetsky, 1965), nor do they appear to be as effective as chlorpromazine in neutralizing reticular stimulation (Kornetsky and Eliasson, 1970). Phenothiazines like promethazine, which have sedative without antipsychotic effects, have not been tested, and such experiments would seem very worthwhile. It is also not known whether tolerance develops to these effects, or whether they are antagonized by anticholinergics.

Self-Stimulation
Self-stimulation through electrodes implanted in the medial forebrain bundle is suppressed by neuroleptics, and this phenomenon satisfies the first isomorphism criterion very well, according to data obtained in rats by Dresse and displayed in Table 2.2. The first column gives the ED_{50} for response suppression (Dresse, 1966), while the second lists the dose of each drug regarded as clinically equivalent to 100 mg chlorpromazine

Table 2.2
Effect of antipsychotic drugs on self-stimulation

	ED_{50}(mg/kg)	Dose equivalent to 100 mg chlorpromazine (mg)
Chlorpromazine	2.0	100.
Prochlorperazine	0.73	14.3
Fluphenazine	0.08	1.2
Chlorprothixene	0.95	43.9
Haloperidol	0.052	1.6

Source: Dresse, 1966.

(Davis, 1974). The correlation coefficient between the clinical and experimental potencies is surprisingly high (r = 0.98).

It would be most interesting to compare the effects of nonantipsychotic phenothiazines on the suppression of self-stimulation and to test for the development of tolerance. The fourth criterion is less favorable: the anticholinergic scopolamine does antagonize chlorpromazine's effect (Olds, 1972). It would also be valuable to study the effects of these drugs on self-stimulation elicited from other intracranial sites. Self-stimulation can be obtained from regions containing cell bodies of the nigrostriatal (Routtenberg and Malsbury, 1969) and mesolimbic (Crow and Gillbe, 1974) dopamine tracts, as well as from the nucleus accumbens septi, which is rich in dopaminergic endings (Fibiger and Phillips, 1974), although it is still controversial whether dopaminergic neurons participate in self-stimulation behavior (Stein et al., 1974; Breese et al., 1974). The pharmacology of self-stimulation elicited from presumptive dopaminergic sites would be especially interesting in view of the widely discussed hypothesis that dopaminergic pathways are involved in the mechanism of action of tranquilizing drugs (Matthysse, 1974).

Operant Performance
Phenothiazines affect various aspects of operant behavior, including rate, quality of performance, and the effects of complex schedules of reinforcement. For example, in a mixed fixed-ratio/fixed-interval schedule there is normally a pause in responding during the early phase of the fixed-interval component, and this pause tends not to occur after chlorpromazine has been administered. Unfortunately the effects of

promazine and chlorpromazine are indistinguishable, despite their marked difference in clinical efficacy (Dews, 1958). Performance on a task involving two levers (a "work key" and a "reinforcement key") was disorganized by chlorpromazine, but equally so by promazine, and haloperidol was relatively ineffective (Laties, 1972).

Tolerance development to the effects of phenothiazines on operant performance has been observed in some studies but not in others. In one experiment tolerance did develop over a fifteen-day period to the deficit in fixed-interval responding caused by chlorpromazine (16 mg/kg/day, in dogs) (Waller, 1961). Similarly tolerance was observed to have an effect on fixed-ratio performance in rats over a relatively long time period (112 days at 5 mg/kg/day chlorpromazine) (Ortiz et al., 1971). On the other hand tolerance did not develop over this time period to effects on discrimination learning (Ortiz et al., 1971) or to effects on a classically conditioned response (Dési et al., 1970).

Human operant performance is also impaired by chlorpromazine on a variety of complex tasks, such as digit-symbol substitution, tracking of a moving target, rapid tapping, and tachistoscopic recognition of numbers. These performance deficits all disappear after repetition of the dose (200 mg/day during the first week, 400 mg/day during the second) for a one- or two-week period (Kornetsky et al., 1959).

In general phenothiazines have a detrimental effect on complex performance, but at least one paradigm has been reported in which chlorpromazine causes improvement: training a pigeon to stand still, a behavior which a normal pigeon can manage for about four seconds. Chlorpromazine increased the length of time the pigeon was able to stand still; pentobarbital, on the other hand, reduced it (Blough, 1958). None of the isomorphism criteria has yet been applied to this intriguing behavioral effect.

The literature on disruption of operant behavior by phenothiazines is, on the whole, too heterogeneous to be considered a coherent model system. There is no reason to expect a priori that learning paradigms will be affected by drugs in the same way unless they are strictly comparable in design. To be valuable as models for schizophrenia experiments in animal learning need to be designed in terms of hypotheses concerning the relationship of the learning paradigm to pathological human cognitive processes. We will return to the problem of designing learning experiments later.

Conditioned Avoidance

The suppressant effect of chlorpromazine on conditioned-avoidance responding was one of the first pharmacological effects of the phenothiazines to be described (Courvoisier, 1953). A delay in responding to the cue that signals a forthcoming shock, caused by the locomotor-depressant effects of chlorpromazine, could conceivably be misinterpreted as an inhibition of avoidance behavior since the increased latency would cause the response to be classified as escape rather than avoidance. The avoidance-responding deficit persists, however, when a compensatory increase in the interval between cue and shock is made (Lipper and Kornetsky, 1971). Passive-avoidance responding is also suppressed by chlorpromazine (Iwahara et al., 1968), and the extinction of previously learned active avoidance proceeds more rapidly (Miller et al., 1957; Davis et al., 1961). Locomotor depression would act in the opposite direction in these two paradigms.

Correlations of antipsychotic potency with suppression of conditioned-avoidance responding are favorable with respect to most of the phenothiazines and butyrophenones tested (Cook and Kelleher, 1962; Cook and Catania, 1964; Niemegeers et al., 1969, 1970; Delini-Stula, 1971). As in other paradigms, thioridazine was found to be less active in suppressing conditioned avoidance in the rat than would be expected from its clinical potency (Swinyard et al., 1959; Niemegeers et al., 1969, 1970; Delini-Stula, 1971). In the monkey, on the other hand, the effectiveness of thioridazine in suppressing conditioned avoidance was similar to that of chlorpromazine (Cook and Catania, 1964). The criterion of correlation between clinical and experimental potency has to be applied with careful regard to the possibility of species differences. Simple escape responses, in addition to being blocked only at higher doses of chlorpromazine (Cook and Catania, 1964), show less satisfactory correlations with clinical potency (Plotnikoff, 1963).

The suppression of conditioned-avoidance responding by chlorpromazine shows tolerance after repeated drug administration (Irwin, 1961, 1963; Stone, 1964). A study of cross-tolerance induced in rats by haloperidol to the avoidance-suppressing effects of flupenthixol, however, was negative (Møller Nielsen et al., 1974). Data on anticholinergic blockade of phenothiazine effects using this paradigm are scarce, but antagonism by scopolamine and trihexyphenidyl has been reported (Morpurgo and Theobald, 1964).

Phenothiazine drugs also suppress social-avoidance behavior, which is of interest because autistic behavior in schizophrenia can be regarded in part as a form of social avoidance. Beagles that have been exposed to isolation stress behave more normally in a social situation when treated with chlorpromazine (Fuller and Clark, 1966). Ewes will normally not accept orphan lambs after they have nursed their own offspring, but a single dose of perphenazine appears to overcome the initial rejection and lead to permanent acceptance of the orphan by the foster mother (Neathery, 1971). Whether social avoidance is equivalent pharmacologically to the simpler avoidance paradigms that have been discussed, or expresses qualitatively different phenomena, is not known.

Other Paradigms

A few additional paradigms have been examined from a comparative pharmacological point of view. Aggression can be provoked in animals in a variety of ways: social isolation, aversive electric shock, lesions in several brain regions (septum, ventromedial hypothalamus, olfactory bulbs). On the whole studies of the inhibition of experimentally induced aggression by phenothiazines show disappointing correlations with clinical potency (Tedeschi et al., 1959; DaVanzo et al., 1966; Sofia, 1969; Malick et al., 1969; Malick, 1970; Funderburk et al., 1970).

Striking behavioral aberrations can be induced in animals by the use of psychotomimetic drugs such as LSD, ranging from the spinning of disordered webs by spiders (Witt, 1958) to a reaction in rats consisting of "piloerection, mydriasis . . . aimless sniffing . . . incessant head movements from side to side . . . compulsive licking and chewing . . . tendency to bite or gnaw the wire mesh floor of the cage . . . reduced pelvic elevation . . . rearing on the hind legs and facing the other animal" (Dixon, 1968). There are very few studies on the antagonism of psychotomimetic-drug-induced abnormal behavior patterns by phenothiazines. In the last-mentioned example several antipsychotic drugs (including thioridazine) inhibited the behavior, but the range of drugs tested was not complete. Reduction of the lethality of toxic doses of mescaline by phenothiazines has been studied comparatively, but correlations with clinical potency were not encouraging (Plotnikoff and Washington, 1958).

Although the experimental data available to test these behavioral models in terms of the isomorphism criteria are far from complete, the studies that have been reviewed show that none of the extant models fares particularly well. That isomorphism with schizophrenia is not present should not surprise us since none of the studies was devised with that purpose in mind. We would now like to propose certain principles for constructing animal models which may increase their likelihood of satisfying the criteria.

1. *Evaluate behavior in the context of the social situation and the animal's repertoire.* The hallmark of psychotic behavior is inappropriateness of response. The response itself may be normal in proper context, but it becomes abnormal in the wrong setting. Embracing, for example, is a perfectly appropriate response when meeting a close friend, but it is inappropriate in Western cultures when one is faced with a stranger or an enemy. Expressing an affect such as laughter at a funeral would be considered equally bizarre. A single response is not sufficient to identify a particular psychotic syndrome; diagnosis requires an internally consistent series of inappropriate behaviors that are regularly evoked in definable contexts. Theories of etiology and therapy rest upon isolating identifiable syndromes of inappropriate behavior, but behavior can only be regarded as aberrant relative to the context of the situation in which it occurs and the range of the animal's repertoire.

To pursue this approach one must have a thorough naturalistic understanding of the observed animal's behavior, for the significance of a given act may otherwise be easily misinterpreted. Certain birds, for example, perform acts when threatening and fighting that seem not to belong to aggressive behavior patterns. Male skylarks will at times stop during an aggressive interaction and peck at the ground as if they were eating; other birds in the same circumstances will preen their feathers, while still others will suddenly put their bills under their scapulars and act as if they were going to sleep (Tinbergen, 1971). When several male baboons are sitting in close proximity to one another, yawning is more likely to indicate a tense situation than to be a sign of boredom (Hall and DeVore, 1965). In primates, laboratory and field responses may differ according to the particular ecological niche from which the animal comes. Urban rhesus, for example, tend to be aggressive toward strange animals and attack, while forest rhesus tend to be conciliatory (Singh, 1969). Some behaviors may seem abnormal which when viewed in context are not. Male langurs, coming in contact with a bisexual group, may attempt to kill or injure the entire infant population of the group (Yoshiba, 1968). It would be necessary to understand the situations in which this behavior takes place in order to decide whether the animal has, in fact, "gone mad." It is thus likely to be more productive to study analogues of pathological changes in human behavior within the context of an animal's natural responses than to seek states that mimic the manifest behavior of the human psychotic.

2. *Balance naturalness and control in the design of the experimental environment.* This approach requires designing an environment where the animal is relatively free to exercise his natural repertoire of behavior, especially his social interactions and cognitive capabilities. The primate is especially valuable for this purpose because of the similarity of his brain structure to that of man, his complex cognitive capabilities, and his rich social interactions. Since environmental stimulation is necessary to maintain a healthy monkey, it is important to provide both a satisfactory physical environment and adequate social stimulation.

An ideal environmental design would encompass an area large enough for relatively free movement and social interaction while still allowing the experimenter the control needed for manipulating the independent variables. On the other hand, in a completely free environment there is the danger of losing contact with the animal, which would abruptly curtail the observations and prevent acquisition of crucial follow-up data (e.g., histological and biochemical measurements). In an unrestricted environment the experimenter's ability to control variables and isolate specific effects and responses would be limited.

3. *Define psychopathology in cross-species terms.* Insofar as psychosis in man is defined exclusively in terms of private thoughts, fantasies, and feelings, it is not possible to study its equivalent in another species (but,

strictly speaking, it cannot be studied in another person either). Psychosis also manifests itself in outward behavior, however, and it is in fact the abnormality of the psychotic's behavior that usually leads to hospitalization. In constructing operational definitions for animal models of psychosis, one should therefore emphasize the behavioral and interactive aspects of psychotic states, and the terms in which psychosis is defined will thus be inherently cross-species. Paranoia and thought disorder will be discussed as examples.

Paranoia   Human paranoia may be thought of as involving three phases: (1) denial of one's own hostility; (2) attribution of hostility to others when it is actually not present; (3) vigilance, social avoidance, and elaboration of delusions. While we have no way to detect denial and delusion formation in animals, it may be possible to study the attribution of hostility to others, as well as the resulting vigilance and social avoidance.

Primates have rich and complicated repertoires of facial expressions and gestures ranging from threatening to neutral and submissive (Hinde and Rowell, 1962; Van Hooff, 1967) and will respond to each other accordingly. Miller, for example, required two *Macaca mulatta* to communicate with each other via facial expression in order to avoid a shock. One animal was able to see the warning light but had no control over the lever that forestalled the shock. The other animal had access to the shock-control lever but could not see the warning light. This animal could, however, see the other, and, by detecting the anxiety in his partner, he learned when to press the lever to avoid the shock for both (Miller et al., 1967). Ability to distinguish facial expressions and gestures could be used as a measure of the correctness of the monkey's perception of social cues and as a basis for studies of the tendency to attribute hostility to other animals when it is not present.

Associative Thought Disorder   It is natural to assume that, since man is the only species with language, he alone can exhibit thought disorder and that this central aspect of schizophrenia can therefore not be studied in animals. Although the most obvious manifestations of thought disorder in humans are expressed through language, we may be able to extract its nonlinguistic characteristics in such a way that an analogy will be applicable to animals. Some of the relevant features include (1) loss of the "abstract attitude"; (2) idiosyncratic responses; (3) inappropriate overgeneralizations from limited aspects of a similar situation. We will consider the first of these.

Abstract conceptualization, although most highly developed in man, is not unique to him. From the classic learning studies of Nissen (1951), French (1965), Robinson (1960), and Bernstein (1961), it has become clear that laboratory monkeys and apes are capable of a sophisticated level of abstraction. For example, rhesus perform well on tasks that require differentiating stimuli on the conceptual basis of oddity. After having been trained to select the odd member of an otherwise identical group, they are able to transfer the concept of oddity to another set of objects, even if the common property (color, shape, size, etc.) in the new group is different from the one used in the original discrimination task.

Chimpanzees are capable of sophisticated levels of abstraction, as demonstrated by their facility in the use of American sign language. Not only are they able to use the signs correctly, but they can also express their own wishes—"tickle me"—and, even more remarkable, can make up their own words—"water-bird" for duck (Gardner and Gardner, 1971). A growing literature from field studies indicates the cleverness of nonhuman primates in manipulation of the environment. Chimps using leaves for sponges and sticks to extract termites are good examples (Van Lawick-Goodall, 1973). In summary it may be possible to construct more satisfactory animal models of psychosis by concentrating on the nonlinguistic operational aspects of psychotic states whose applicability is not confined to man.

4. *Model human psychoses of known etiology and predictable symptoms.* It would be helpful in constructing an animal model to have in mind a form of human psychosis with a known etiology which can be reliably induced by some manipulation (either biological or environmental). If the manipulation produces variable effects in man with no predictability, the associated animal model will be confusing. For example, many brain syndromes associated with poisons (e.g., bromides) or lesions in the central nervous system (e.g., temporal-lobe epilepsy) may produce personality changes, but the effects are variable and there are a variety of symptoms that may or may not be present.

Unfortunately there are very few psychosis-inducing agents that meet the criterion of reliability. Amphetamine is relatively reliable in producing paranoia in man, but the dose and time required varies with the individual. Separation trauma is fairly consistent in eliciting depression, and LSD predictably produces hallucinations (among other symptoms). A cross-species test for abnormal mental functioning can be most easily devised using an agent that reliably produces this disturbance in man. The same test might later be applied to animal behavioral abnormalities whose etiology is less clear.

In conclusion we suggest that *nonlinguistic* operational definitions of human psychosis be taken as the starting point for constructing animal models so that the definitions will be inherently applicable across species. It is likely that even "higher" aspects of psychosis in man, such as paranoia and loss of the abstract attitude, may have equivalents in animals if they are formulated in nonlinguistic terms. Ultimately these models can be tested, not only by their resemblance to aspects of schizophrenia, but also by their pharmacological sensitivities. Parallelism in the reaction to tranquilizing drugs *(isomorphism)* may indicate that there is an underlying homology between the brain structures that subserve the animal behavior and the structures in man that are implicated in schizophrenia.

References

Arnfred, T., and Randrup, A. 1968. Cholinergic mechanism in brain inhibiting amphetamine-induced stereotyped behaviour. *Acta Pharmacol. Toxicol.* (Kbh) 26:384–394.

Asper, H., Baggiolini, M., Burki, H. R., Lauener, H., Ruch, W., and Stille, G. 1973. Tolerance phenomena with neuroleptics: Catalepsy, apomorphine stereotypies and striatal dopamine metabolism in the rat after single and repeated administration of loxapine and haloperidol. *Eur. J. Pharmacol.* 22:287–294.

Barnett, A., Goldstein, J., and Taber, R. I. 1972. Apomorphine-induced hypothermia in mice: A possible dopaminergic effect. *Arch. Int. Pharmacodyn. Ther.* 198:242–247.

Bernstein, I. S. 1961. The utilization of visual cues in dimension-abstracted oddity by primates. *J. Comp. Physiol. Psychol.* 54:243–247.

Blough, D. S. 1958. New test for tranquilizers. *Science* 127:586–587.

Boyd, E. M. 1960. Chlorpromazine tolerance and physical dependence. *J. Pharmacol. Exp. Ther.* 128:75–78.

Breese, G. R., Cooper, B. R. and Hollister, A. S. 1974. Relationship of biogenic amines to behavior. In S. Matthysse and S. S. Kety, eds., *Catecholamines and their enzymes in the neuropathology of schizophrenia.* Oxford: Pergamon.

Cook, L., and Catania, A. C. 1964. Effects of drugs on avoidance and escape behavior. *Fed. Proc.* 23:818–835.

Cook, L., and Kelleher, R. T. 1962. Drug effects on the behavior of animals. *Ann. N.Y. Acad. Sci.* 96:315–335.

Cook, L., Weidley, E., Deegan, J., and Mattis, P. A. 1958. Evaluation of a group of centrally acting agents. *J. Pharmacol. Exp. Ther.* 122:14–15.

Courvoisier, S. 1953. Propriétés pharmacodynamiques du chlorhydrate de chloro-3(diméthylamino-3'propyl)-10 phénothiazine (4.560 R.P.): Étude experimentale d'un nouveau corps utilisé dans l'anesthésie potentialisée et dans l'hibernation artificielle. *Arch. Int. Pharmacodyn. Ther.* 92:305–361.

Crow, T. J., and Gillbe, C. 1974. Brain dopamine and behaviour. In S. Matthysse and S. S. Kety, eds., *Catecholamines and their enzymes in the neuropathology of schizophrenia.* Oxford: Pergamon.

DaVanzo, J. P., Daugherty, M., Ruckart, R., and Kang, L. 1966. Pharmacological and biochemical studies in isolation-induced fighting mice. *Psychopharmacologia* 9:210–219.

Davis, J. M. 1974. Dose equivalence of the anti-psychotic drugs. In S. Matthysse and S. S. Kety, eds., *Catecholamines and their enzymes in the neuropathology of schizophrenia.* Oxford: Pergamon.

Davis, W. M., Capehart, T., and Llewellin, W. L. 1961. Mediated acquisitions of a fear-motivated response and inhibitory effects of chlorpromazine. *Psychopharmacologia* 2:268–276.

Delini-Stula, A. 1971. Drug-induced suppression of conditioned hyperthermic and conditioned avoidance behavior response in rats. *Psychopharmacologia* 20:153–159.

Dési, I., Kertai, P., Farkas, I., Muskó, Zs., and Hajós, P. 1970. The process of learning in rats undergoing prolonged treatment with psychotropic agents. *Psychopharmacologia* 18:144–153.

Dews, P. B. 1958. Effects of chlorpromazine and promazine on performance on a mixed schedule of reinforcement. *J. Exp. Anal. Behav.* 1:73–82.

Dixon, A. K. 1968. Evidence of catecholamine mediation in the "aberrant" behavior induced by lysergic acid diethylamide (LSD) in the rat. *Experientia* 24:743–747.

Dresse, A. 1966. Influence de 15 neuroleptiques (butyrophénones et phénothiazines) sur les variations de la teneur du cerveau en noradrénaline et l'activité du rat dans le test d'autostimulation. *Arch. Int. Pharmacodyn. Ther.* 159:353–365.

Ellinwood, E. H., Jr., Sudilovsky, A., and Nelson, L. M. 1973. Evolving behavior in the clinical and experimental amphetamine (model) psychosis. *Am. J. Psychiatry* 130:1088–1093.

Fibiger, H. C., and Phillips, A. G. 1974. The role of dopamine and norepinephrine in the chemistry of reward. In S. Matthysse and S. S. Kety, eds., *Catecholamines and their enzymes in the neuropathology of schizophrenia.* Oxford: Pergamon.

Fjalland, B., and Møller Nielsen, I. 1974. Methylphenidate antagonism of haloperidol, interaction with cholinergic and anticholinergic drugs. *Psychopharmacologia* 34:111–118.

French, G. M. 1965. Associative problems. In A. M. Schrier, H. F. Harlow, and F. Stollwitz, eds., *Behavior of nonhuman primates.* New York: Academic Press.

Fuller, J. L., and Clark, L. D. 1966. Genetic and treatment factors modifying the postisolation syndrome in dogs. *J. Comp. Physiol. Psychol.* 61:251–257.

Funderburk, W. H., Foxwell, M. H., and Hakala, M. W. 1970. Effects of psychotherapeutic drugs on hypothalamic-induced hissing in cats. *Neuropharmacology* 9:1–7.

Gardner, B. T., and Gardner, A. 1971. Two-way communication with an infant chimpanzee. In A. Schrier and F. Stollwitz, eds., *Behavior of nonhuman primates.* New York: Academic Press.

Gupta, G. P., and Dhawan, B. N. 1965. Blockade of apomorphine pecking with phenothiazines. *Psychopharmacologia* 8:120–130.

Hall, K. R. L., and DeVore, I. 1965. Baboon social behavior. In I. DeVore, ed., *Primate behavior: Field studies of monkeys and apes.* New York: Holt, Rinehart and Winston.

Hinde, R. A., and Rowell, T. E. 1962. Communication by postures and facial expressions in the rhesus monkey (*Macaca mulatta*). *Proc. Zool. Soc. Lond.* 138:1–21.

Irwin, S. 1961. Correlation in rats between the locomotor and avoidance suppressant potencies of eight phenothiazine tranquilizers. *Arch. Int. Pharmacodyn. Ther.* 132:279–286.

Irwin, S. 1963. Influence of external factors and arousal mechanisms on the rate of drug tolerance development. *Arch. Int. Pharmacodyn. Ther.* 142:152–162.

Iwahara, S., Iwasaki, T., and Hasegawa, Y. 1968. Effects of chlorpromazine and homofenazine upon a passive avoidance response in rats. *Psychopharmacologia* 13:320–331.

Janssen, P. S. J., Niemegeers, C. J. E., Schellekens, H. K. L., and Lenaerts, F. M. 1967. Is it possible to predict the clinical effects of neuroleptic drugs (major tranquilizers) from animal data? IV. An improved experimental design for measuring the inhibitory effects of neuroleptic drugs on amphetamine- or apomorphine-induced "Cheroing" and "agitation" in rats. *Arzneim. Forsch.* 17:841–854.

Klawans, H. L., and Rubovits, R. 1972. An experimental model of tardive dyskinesia. *J. Neural Transmission* 33:235–246.

Kornetsky, C., and Bain, G. 1965. The effects of chlorpromazine and pentobarbital on sustained attention in the rat. *Psychopharmacologia* 8:277-284.

Kornetsky, C., and Eliasson, M. 1969. Reticular stimulation and chlorpromazine: An animal model for schizophrenic overarousal. *Science* 165:1273-1274.

Kornetsky, C., and Eliasson, M. 1970. Reticular stimulation and chlorpromazine. *Science* 168:1123.

Kornetsky, C., Petit, M., Wynne, R., and Evarts, E. 1959. A comparison of the psychological effects of acute and chronic administration of chlorpromazine and secobarbital (quinalbarbitone) in chronic schizophrenic patients. *J. Ment. Sci.* 105:190-198.

Laties, V. G. 1972. The modification of drug effects on behavior by external discriminative stimuli. *J. Pharmacol. Exp. Ther.* 183:1-13.

Latz, A., and Kornetsky, C. 1965. The effects of chlorpromazine and secobarbital under two conditions of reinforcement on the performance of chronic schizophrenic subjects. *Psychopharmacologia* 7:77-88.

Lipper, S., and Kornetsky, C. 1971. Effect of chlorpromazine on conditioned avoidance as a function of CS-US interval length. *Psychopharmacologia* 22:144-150.

Malick, J. B. 1970. Effects of selected drugs on stimulus-bound emotional behavior elicited by hypothalamic stimulation in the cat. *Arch. Int. Pharmacodyn. Ther.* 186:137-141.

Malick, J. B., Sofia, R. D., and Goldberg, M. E. 1969. A comparative study of the effects of selected psychoactive agents upon three lesion-induced models of aggression in the rat. *Arch. Int. Pharmacodyn. Ther.* 181:459-465.

Matthysse, S. 1973. Antipsychotic drug actions: A clue to the neuropathology of schizophrenia? *Fed. Proc.* 5:200-205.

Matthysse, S. 1974. Implications of catecholamine systems of the brain in schizophrenia. In F. Plum, ed., *Brain dysfunction in metabolic disorders.* New York: Raven Press.

Miller, R. E., Caul, W. F., and Mirsky, I. A. 1967. Communication of affects between feral and socially isolated monkeys. *J. Pers. Soc. Psychol.* 7:231-239.

Miller, R. E., Murphy, J. V., and Mirsky, I. A. 1957. The effect of chlorpromazine on fear-motivated behavior in rats. *J. Pharmacol. Exp. Ther.* 120:379-387.

Mirsky, A. F., and Bloch, S. 1967. Effects of chlorpromazine, secobarbital and sleep deprivation on attention in monkeys. *Psychopharmacologia* 10:388-399.

Møller Nielsen, I., Fjalland, B., Pedersen, V., and Nymark, M. 1974. Pharmacology of neuroleptics upon repeated administration. *Psychopharmacologia* 34:95-104.

Morpurgo, C., and Theobald, W. 1964. Influence of antiparkinson drugs and amphetamine on some pharmacological effects of phenothiazine derivatives used as neuroleptics. *Psychopharmacologia* 6:178-191.

Neathery, M. W. 1971. Acceptance of orphan lambs by tranquilized ewes (*Ovis aries*). *Anim. Behav.* 19:75–79.

Niemegeers, C. J. E., Verbruggen, F. J., and Janssen, P. A. J. 1969. The influence of various neuroleptic drugs on shock avoidance responding in rats. I. Nondiscriminated Sidman avoidance procedure. II. Nondiscriminated Sidman avoidance precedure with alternate reinforcement and extinction periods and analysis of the interresponse times (IRT's). *Psychopharmacologia* 16:161–174.

Niemegeers, C. J. E., Verbruggen, F. J., and Janssen, P. A. J. 1970. The influence of various neuroleptic drugs on noise escape response in rats. *Psychopharmacologia* 18:249–259.

Nissen, H. W. 1951. Analysis of a complex conditional reaction in chimpanzee. *J. Comp. Physiol. Psychol.* 44:9.

Olds, M. E. 1972. Alterations by centrally acting drugs of the suppression of self-stimulation behavior in the rat by tetrabenazine, physostigmine, chlorpromazine and pentobarbital. *Psychopharmacologia* 25:299–314.

Ortiz, A., Glover, A., and Lang, W. J. 1971. The effects of acute and chronic administration of chlorpromazine on the acquisition and extinction of positively reinforced operant responses. *Physiol. Behav.* 6:407–412.

Plotnikoff, N. P. 1963. Effect of neurotropic drugs on a non-conditioned avoidance response. *Arch. Int. Pharmacodyn. Ther.* 145:430–439.

Plotnikoff, N. P., and Washington, H. 1958. Bioassay of ataractics against lethal action of mescaline in mice. *Proc. Soc. Exp. Biol. Med.* 98:660–662.

Randrup, A. 1974. Pharmacology and physiology of stereotyped behavior. In S. Matthysse and S. S. Kety, eds., *Catecholamines and their enzymes in the neuropathology of schizophrenia.* Oxford: Pergamon.

Robinson, J. S. 1960. The conceptual basis of the chimpanzee's performance on the sameness-difference discrimination problem. *J. Comp. Physiol. Psychol.* 53:368–370.

Rotrosen, J., Wallach, M. B., Angrist, B., and Gershon, S. 1972. Antagonism of apomorphine-induced stereotypy and emesis in dogs by thioridazine, haloperidol and pimozide. *Psychopharmacologia* 26:185–194.

Routtenberg, A., and Malsbury, C. 1969. Brainstem pathways of reward. *J. Comp. Physiol. Psychol.* 68:22–30.

Rowell, T. 1972. *Social behavior of monkeys.* Baltimore: Penguin.

Senault, B. 1970. Comportement d'agressivité intraspécifique induit par l'apomorphine chez le rat. *Psychopharmacologia* 18:271–287.

Shillito, E. E. 1967. The effect of chlorpromazine and thioridazine on the exploration of a Y-maze by rats. *Br. J. Pharmacol.* 30:258–264.

Singh, M. M., and Smith, J. M. 1973. Reversal of some therapeutic effects of an antipsychotic agent by an antiparkinsonism drug. *J. Nerv. Ment. Dis.* 157:50–58.

Singh, S. D. 1969. Urban monkeys. *Sci. Am.* 221:108–115.

Sofia, R. D. 1969. Effects of centrally active drugs on four models of experimentally-induced aggression in rodents. *Life Sci.* [I] 8:705–716.

Stein, L., Belluzzi, J. D., Ritter, S., and Wise, C. D. 1974. Self-stimulation reward pathways: Norepinephrine vs. dopamine. In S. Matthysse and S. S. Kety, eds., *Catecholamines and their enzymes in the neuropathology of schizophrenia.* Oxford: Pergamon.

Stone, G. C. 1964. Dosing order and depression of avoidance behavior by chlorpromazine. *Psychol. Rep.* 15:175–178.

Swinyard, E. A., Wolf, H. H., Fink, G. B., and Goodman, L. S. 1959. Some neuropharmacological properties of thioridazine hydrochloride (Mellaril). *J. Pharmacol. Exp. Ther.* 126:312–317.

Tedeschi, R. E., Tedeschi, D. H., Mucha, H., Cook, L., Mattis, P. A., and Fellows, E. J. 1959. Effects of various centrally acting drugs on fighting behavior of mice. *J. Pharmacol. Exp. Ther.* 125:28–34.

Tinbergen, N. 1971. *Herring gull's world.* New York: Harper & Row.

Van Lawick-Goodall, J. 1973. The behavior of chimpanzees in their natural habitat. *Am. J. Psychiatry* 130:1–12.

Van Hooff, J. A. R. A. M. 1967. The facial displays of the catarrhine monkeys and apes. In D. Morris, ed., *Primate ethology.* Chicago: Aldine.

Vencovsky, E. 1967. Antipsychoticke pusobeni thiethylperazinu a klinicke zkusenosti s jeho aplikaci v psychiatrii. *Cesk. Psychiatr.* 63:1–8.

Waller, M. B. 1961. Effects of chronically administered chlorpromazine on multiple-schedule performance. *J. Exp. Anal. Behav.* 4:351–359.

Wilson, M. C., and Schuster, C. R. 1972. The effects of chlorpromazine on psychomotor stimulant self-administration in the Rhesus monkey. *Psychopharmacologia* 26:115–126.

Witt, P. N. 1958. The identification of small quantities of hallucinatory substances in body fluids with the spider test. In C. F. Reed, I. E. Alexander, and S. S. Tomkins, eds., *Psychopathology: A source book.* Cambridge, Mass.: Harvard.

Yoshiba, K. 1968. Local and intertroop variability in ecology and social behavior of common Indian langurs. In P. Jay, ed., *Primates. Studies in adaptation and variability.* New York: Holt, Rinehart and Winston.

3

Animal Models and Schizophrenia

Conan Kornetsky and Robert Markowitz

Direct animal models have been developed for many human disease states such as hypertension, cancer, and diabetes. Using such models, researchers have been able to uncover much information concerning the underlying mechanisms of these disease states. This has been possible because in these cases the close similarities between the animal and human states have fostered an assurance that the researcher's experimental manipulations will have a direct parallel in man.

In the field of mental illness we are not quite so fortunate. It is possible, as the terminology implies, that mental illness is a uniquely human disorder. With schizophrenia, unlike those diseases mentioned above, it is often difficult to determine the particular variables that define the disease. Certainly animals can be made to behave in a manner that appears to the human observer to be depressed, anxious, fearful, or aggressive. In some cases, however, these descriptions may be more in the eye of the beholder than in the brain of the animal, for we do often tend to attribute our own human experience to animals. Conversely, while a phenomenon such as aggression is amenable to animal modeling, certain types of behavior may be so uniquely human that they cannot be meaningfully replicated in animals. Could we, for example, develop an animal model for dishonesty?

If we are to consider animal models for mental illness, it is thus of paramount importance that we attempt to identify those aspects of the disease that are its defining characteristics. As was pointed out in Chapter 2, it is not necessary that the animal model be exactly analogous to the human paradigm; however, from a heuristic point of view,

C. Kornetsky, Division of Psychiatry and Department of Pharmacology, and R. Markowitz, Department of Pharmacology, Boston University School of Medicine, Boston, MA, 02118. Many of the experiments described in this paper were supported by NIMH Grant 12568. CK is recipient of NIMH Career Scientist Award MH 1759.

similarities can be quite helpful. We could, perhaps, teach an animal to wear clothes and then "indecently expose" itself, or to mutilate itself (behaviors seen in the mentally ill human), but it is not at all clear, a priori, that such a model would teach us anything about the etiology and process of mental illness.

In the present chapter we will describe four types of model that have been used in the study of mental disease states: the first is the conditioned-avoidance response, which is a frequently used assay for antipsychotic drugs; the second is drug-induced disruption of behavior, which provides both an animal and a human model of mental illness; the third is based on a hypothesis that schizophrenia involves a deficit in a postulated "reward system"; and the fourth, used in our laboratory, involves an attempt to reproduce in animals a specific attention deficit that appears to be characteristic of some schizophrenics.

The Conditioned-Avoidance Response
Drug houses have an obvious need for a simple animal model that will selectively pick out antipsychotic drugs and hopefully predict their potency. The conditioned-avoidance response (CAR) is the procedure traditionally used for this purpose. An animal is presented with a conditioned stimulus (CS), a buzzer or a bell, which is followed after a predetermined interval by a noxious unconditioned stimulus (UCS) such as a foot shock. A response (lever press, wheel turn, etc.) during the interval between CS and UCS allows the animal to avoid the shock. If the animal fails to avoid the UCS, the same response will then allow him to escape the UCS. Antipsychotic drugs (but not barbiturates or the so-called minor tranquilizers) selectively inhibit avoidance responding while leaving escape responding intact.

This effect has been interpreted in various ways. One simple interpretation is that the drugs in some way depress the "anxiety" generated by the impending foot shock. The problems with this interpretation are: (1) drugs that are supposedly antianxiety agents do not have this selective effect, and (2) well-trained animals do not show evidence of anxiety or fear such as defecation, piloerection, or biting the grid floor. It has also been suggested that the drug effect is simply the result of motor retardation. However, there is little overt evidence of motor retardation, and at appropriate doses escape behavior appears to be unaffected. Drugs such as barbiturates, which are not specifically antipsychotic, suppress avoidance responding only at doses that cause ataxia and equally impair escape behavior. The specific relationship of the CAR to schizophrenia is thus still obscure; however, the model does seem to allow for the prediction of whether or not a drug may have antipsychotic activity.

Drug Models of Psychosis

It appeared to some that the problems inherent in animal models of psychosis had been circumvented when compounds became available that could induce in "normal" humans what was hoped to be a temporary, reversible psychosis. It had long been known that drugs could produce delirium; however, compounds such as LSD and mescaline appeared to be unique in that they could produce delusional states, states of altered affect, and altered consciousness in the presence of an unclouded sensorium. The term "psychotomimetic" was optimistically coined in the fifties (Gerard, 1956) to describe these drugs. The compounds were also exciting from a theoretical point of view because they chemically resemble putative endogenous neurotransmitters. LSD contains the indole nucleus of serotonin, and mescaline is a phenylethylamine similar to norepinephrine and dopamine. As the drug-induced state could perhaps model psychosis, the drugs themselves could model, on a molecular level, a hypothetical biochemical lesion underlying the psychotic state. It was suggested that some aberrant metabolite of an endogenous substance could be the offending compound producing the psychoses. Research has flourished, but to date no convincing data has been provided to substantiate this theory.

The LSD- and mescaline-induced states are currently not in vogue as a model. Their clinical resemblance to true psychosis was challenged as competent psychiatrists became more sophisticated and could readily make the differential diagnosis between an "LSD trip" and "real schizophrenia." Their biochemical relevance was also questioned after reports that tolerance develops to the hallucinogenic properties of LSD. This fact suggests that these compounds are not good candidates for the putative *endogenous* psychotogen that is supposed to underlie a chronic disease state. "Tolerance" apparently does not develop to schizophrenia.

Although these weaknesses in the LSD-mescaline model are important to consider, they do not conclusively negate its value. Some researchers even feel they have found the "aberrant metabolite" in schizophrenic patients (see, for example, Feldstein (1970) and references therein). Schizophrenia is a complicated dynamic phenomenon. That hallucinogens do not exactly mimic it in all respects, or at all times, does not necessarily imply that these drugs are not valid models for some aspects of the disease, or for the disease state at some point in its ontogeny. The questions of tolerance also may not be critical. Perhaps a schizophrenic patient "produces" his endogenous hallucinogen only in response to recurring stimuli such as stress.

Also, although the drug models discussed above are not the current vogue, it is interesting to note that Wyatt and coworkers (1973) have recently described an enzyme found in human blood which is quite capable of converting naturally occurring substances into a potent "psychotomimetic," N,N-dimethyltryptamine. There are many interesting and frustrating methodological problems encountered in the study and testing of drug models of psychosis in humans. For a detailed discussion of the theories and the research problems the reader is referred to Hollister (1968) and Smythies (1970).

A drug model of psychosis that is currently generating much interest (and attention from the lay press) is the amphetamine-induced model psychosis. Unlike the drugs described above, amphetamine in single doses rarely produces a psychosis-like state. However, chronic administration of high doses will regularly induce a state described by some as almost indistinguishable from paranoid schizophrenia (Griffith et al., 1972). Snyder (1973) states:

Because of its close clinical similarity to acute paranoid schizophrenia, amphetamine psychosis may serve as a useful experimental model for schizophrenia. Molecular and clinical studies suggest that both the schizophrenia-like symptoms of amphetamine psychosis and the specific ability of phenothiazines to relieve the symptoms of schizophrenia and amphetamine psychosis may be the result of interactions with dopamine systems in the brain.

The molecular evidence that dopamine is the relevant putative neurotransmitter is based in part on an assumption that noradrenergic systems, because of the stereospecificity of their receptor sites, will differentiate between d- and l-amphetamine to a much greater extent than will dopaminergic systems; that is, in behavioral systems where d- and l-amphetamine are approximately equipotent it is assumed that dopamine is the neurotransmitter mediating the drug effect. There is considerable evidence to support this assumption (Snyder, 1973); however, it is not universally accepted. Pharmacological investigations (see Chapter 2) further implicate dopamine as a neurotransmitter important in schizophrenia. Of particular relevance to this chemical model is the observation that d- and l-amphetamine are approximately equipotent in their ability to induce the "model psychosis," whereas the dextro form is significantly more potent than the levo form in producing generalized arousal in both humans and animals. In animals d- and l-amphetamine at roughly equivalent doses will regularly induce stereotyped behavior, which may include repetitive grooming, licking, gnawing, head turning, or sniffing. The particular type of behavior elicited will depend upon the species tested and may even vary from animal to animal within a given species.

This drug-induced stereotypy is seen by some as a potential animal model for (at least) acute paranoid schizophrenia. There are many superficial similarities between this characteristic animal response to amphetamine and behavior seen in both the "speed freak" and the true paranoid schizophrenic. Some schizophrenics, and normals during periods of chronic amphetamine intoxication, will often repeat (endlessly) apparently aimless behavior such as emptying and refilling a handbag, taking apart and reassembling a radio, sweeping the same floor, unbuttoning and rebuttoning clothes. Head bobbing, continuous although aimless searching, and increased eye scanning are also observed. Ellinwood and coworkers (1972), studying man and lower animals during chronic amphetamine intoxication, have vividly described the formal similarities between animal and human stereotypies.

Pharmacological evidence lends further credence to this model. Those drugs known to show a high specificity as antipsychotics have been the drugs of choice in treating acute and chronic amphetamine "poisoning," and are the most efficacious in blocking or reversing the drug-induced stereotypies in animals.* It is well documented that the antipsychotics, the phenothiazines and butyrophenones, are effective dopaminergic blocking agents. There is also a plethora of neurophysiological evidence implicating brain dopaminergic tracts as mediators of amphetamine-induced stereotypy.

The system most studied has been the nigrostriatal tract. Considering its involvement with the extrapyramidal motor system, the suggested relationship between this dopaminergic system and amphetamine-induced stereotypies is not particularly surprising. However, this system may be providing more of a bioassay than a model. From a neuroanatomical point of view it is not clear how a deficit within the nigrostriatal tract alone could account for the various symptoms seen in paranoid (and other) schizophrenic patients. Fortunately, however, research has more recently provided us with dopaminergic tracts (nuclei) intimately involved with the limbic system. Conceptually these would appear to be more likely candidates as substrates for dysfunction in psychosis and as sites of action for the antipsychotics (see Chapter 6).

Machiyama and coworkers (1970) have studied *chronic* methamphetamine intoxication. Considering that chronic dosing is necessary to produce the psychosis in humans, this would appear to be particularly relevant. Using a variety of behavioral tests in a variety of animals, they were able to alter a wide range of "performances." Unfortunately a consistent "model" common to all did not appear to evolve, and considerable anthropomorphic interpretation was necessary to produce convincing evidence of relevance to schizophrenia. In general Machiyama describes "a decrease in motor activity, especially in locomotion, indifference to the surroundings and an impoverished repertoire of behavior patterns."

In the minds of some the amphetamine model of psychosis has become virtually synonymous with the dopamine model of psychosis. This is inappropriate, however, and may tend to obscure important data.

* A note of caution was added at this symposium; the specificity that the phenothiazines apparently show in blocking the effects of amphetamine intoxication is being questioned on the basis of some new clinical observations.

The documented effects of amphetamine upon noradrenergic and serotonergic systems certainly should not be ignored. Even accepting a critical role for the dopaminergic tracts mediating the amphetamine psychosis, other systems should not be ignored. Bradley's work (Bradley and Key, 1968; Boakes et al., 1972) on a neuronal basis for the alerting by d-amphetamine clearly implicates noradrenergic neurons in the midbrain reticular system. Perhaps what is needed for this drug model of psychosis is stimulation of dopaminergic limbic nuclei *and* sustained, increased arousal with a reduced capacity for selective inattention.

A "Reward-Appreciation-Deficit" Model

Stein and Wise (1971) have proposed a novel theory and model of schizophrenia. They suggest that schizophrenics have a basic deficit in their reward system, and that they cannot appropriately perceive or "appreciate" rewards. Since the original work by Olds and Milner (1954), considerable neurophysiological evidence has accumulated that supports their contention that there is a discrete neuroanatomical "reward system" coursing through the medial forebrain bundle and that the system may be noradrenergic in nature (Crow, 1973, 1972; Stein, 1964). Stein and Wise postulate the existence of an enzyme defect that allows for the accumulation, at the noradrenergic nerve terminals, of a highly toxic substance (6-hydroxydopamine) that destroys the nerves. They further suggest that the antipsychotic agents exert their beneficial effects by protecting the noradrenergic nerves in the reward system from the destructive effects of 6-hydroxydopamine.

In order to test this theory in animals Wise and Stein administered 6-hydroxydopamine directly into the ventricles of experimental animals. Among the behavioral deficits seen was a decrease in self-stimulatory behavior, which was interpreted to reflect damage in the reward pathways and was felt to model the proposed deficit in schizophrenics. One argument against this aspect of the model is that, apparently, a priming dose of electrical stimulation (that is, a noncontingent stimulus delivered by the experimenter) can restore the animals' self-stimulatory behavior. This would be consistent with a decrease in the level of arousal due to the experimental drug rather than a decrease in the animals' ability to appreciate rewarding stimuli per se.

Given large doses of 6-hydroxydopamine, the animals show a type of immobility described as "waxy flexibility." Wise and Stein suggest that this may also model a behavioral phenomenon seen in some schizophrenics. It should be noted in this connection, however, that, depending particularly upon the time after dosage, animals treated with 6-hydroxydopamine may appear very sick in a nonspecific way.

There are many weaknesses to the model Wise and Stein propose, but it is of great heuristic value. (For further discussion see the series of letters published in *Science* 175:919–923.)

A Neuropsychological Model

Thus far, models of schizophrenia that have attempted to produce schizophrenia-like behavior by means of drugs have been emphasized. This section will deal with our attempt to develop a model that has relevance to the schizophrenic process by provoking in animals a behavioral deficit similar to one seen in some schizophrenics. The idea of this animal model did not appear suddenly, but was slowly developed from a series of observations in patients and normal controls. Our strategy was to develop for animals procedures and techniques that would mimic, in part, the behavior of patients and the response of patients to drugs.

As noted above, the first task is to determine which of the many behavioral deficits exhibited by schizophrenic patients are primary manifestations of the disease. Work in our laboratory has suggested that the "core" deficit, at least in some schizophrenics, involves an impairment in simple attention. Experiments with patients have led to the hypothesis that some schizophrenics are in a state of chronic central hyperarousal which is the result of a dysfunction of those parts of the central nervous system that subserve the maintenance of arousal and attention—that is, the mesencephalic reticular formation.

Two psychological tests have figured prominently in the development of our thoughts about schizophrenia. The continuous performance test (CPT) was originally developed by Rosvold and coworkers (1965) as a measure of brain damage. In one form it consists of visual stimuli, such as letters, presented to subjects for 0.1 second with a 1.0-second interstimulus interval. One letter is designated as the "critical stimulus," and it appears, on the average, one out of every six or seven presentations. The order of presentation is random. The subject's task is to press a key within the 1.1-second response time after the appearance of the critical stimulus. Two types of error are possible in this test: error of commission and error of omission. An error of commission occurs when the subject presses the key in response to a noncritical stimulus, and an error of omission occurs when the subject fails to respond to the critical stimulus (see Figure 3.1). The digit-symbol substitution test (DSST) is a subtest of the Wechsler Test of Adult Intelligence and is a good predictor of the overall test score. The DSST requires a brief, usually 90-second, cognitive effort, while the CPT requires a slightly

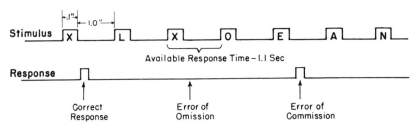

Figure 3.1 An example of the time sequence and types of error on the CPT. Adapted from Kornetsky (1972).

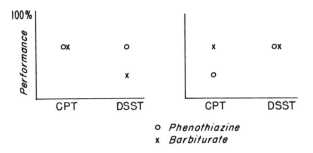

Figure 3.2 The graph on the left is a schematic illustration of the case where doses of a phenothiazine and a barbiturate that cause equal impairment of performance on the CPT differentially affect performance on the DSST, with the barbiturate causing the greater impairment. The graph on the right depicts the converse situation where doses that are equipotent with regard to the DSST differentially affect performance on the CPT, the phenothiazine causing the greater impairment.

longer effort, usually 4 to 8 minutes, of sustained attention. Brief lapses of attention will be manifest as errors of omission on the CPT, whereas such lapses will only affect DSST performance if they are very extensive.

The CPT and DSST appear to respond to alterations in different neural systems or substrates. For example, sleep deprivation and petit mal epilepsy both impair performance on the CPT. The phenothiazines and the barbiturates, two classes of drugs capable of differentially altering central-nervous-system activity, will differentially alter performance on the two tests (Mirsky and Kornetsky, 1964). Those drugs which act at higher cortical levels, such as low doses of barbiturates (Brazier, 1973), seem to affect performance on the DSST selectively. If doses of chlorpromazine and secobarbital are chosen that cause equivalent impairment on the DSST, these doses will differentially impair performance on the CPT, with chlorpromazine causing the greater impairment. Using doses of the two drugs that cause equal impairment on the CPT, the barbiturate will cause greater impairment of performance on the DSST than will the phenothiazine (see Figure 3.2). (The figure we present here is a schematic, for we can rarely get equivalent doses.) Neurophysiological and behavioral evidence relating to this pharmacological dissociation has been discussed by Mirsky and Kornetsky (1964).

In summary the evidence suggests that the chlorpromazine effect is more pronounced on a task measuring sustained attention (CPT) because chlorpromazine acts on the midbrain and brain-stem structures that mediate arousal, whereas the barbiturate effect is more pronounced on a task measuring cognitive ability (DSST) because the primary action of moderate doses of this drug is on the cortex.

In an attempt to duplicate this drug-induced dissociation phenomenon in animals we devised the following test situation. In place of the "letter" stimuli used in the human CPT, two lights were placed in the test chamber, one above the other (Kornetsky and Bain, 1965). (See Figure 3.3.) To parallel the human test one light was designated the critical and the other the noncritical stimulus. Stimuli were presented in a pseudorandom fashion, the ratio of critical to noncritical being approximately 1:6. The stimuli were presented for 0.2 seconds, with an available response time of 3 seconds between presentations. The animal,

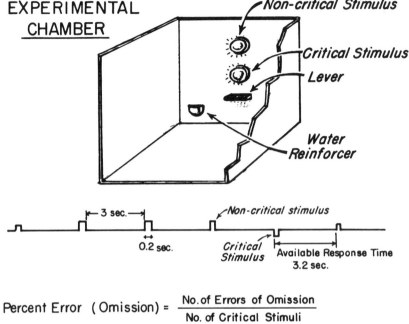

Figure 3.3. An animal version of the CPT. From Kornetsky and Bain (1965).

$$\text{Percent Error (Omission)} = \frac{\text{No. of Errors of Omission}}{\text{No. of Critical Stimuli}}$$

$$\text{Percent Error (Commission)} = \frac{\text{No. of Responses to Non-critical Stimulus}}{\text{No. of Critical Stimuli}}$$

in this case a rat, was trained on a simple go/no-go task. A lever press following the presentation of a critical stimulus was followed by a water reinforcement. Failure to respond to a critical stimulus (error of omission) or a response to a noncritical stimulus (error of commission) had no consequence. As can be seen from Figures 3.4 and 3.5, chlorpromazine caused a monotonic increase in errors of omission as a function of dose, with little systematic change in commission errors. On the other hand pentobarbital, with the exception of the highest dose used, caused the opposite effect. The results of this experiment clearly suggest that the procedure with the rat is analogous to that used in man.

Returning to the human studies, it is appropriate to discuss our thoughts about the specific relevance of the above studies to schizophrenia. It has been suggested by a number of investigators (Venables and Wing, 1962; Venables, 1964; Blum, 1957; Hill, 1957) that there may be some primary dysfunction in the arousal system, and the subcortical areas that subserve arousal, in the schizophrenic patient. On the basis of a wide diversity of evidence Kornetsky and Mirsky (1966) concluded that in some schizophrenics there may be a malfunction in the midbrain or brain-stem reticular formation. An altered arousal system could account for much of the impairment seen in the schizophrenic and, more specifically, for the patient's inability to maintain a "set" in the reaction-time experiments of Shakow (1962) and others (Fedio et al., 1961; Venables, 1964).

Orzack and Kornetsky (1966) studied chronic schizophrenics, patients in treatment for chronic alcoholism, and normal volunteers, using the CPT and the DSST. The schizophrenics had been off medication for at least three months prior to study, and the alcoholics had been

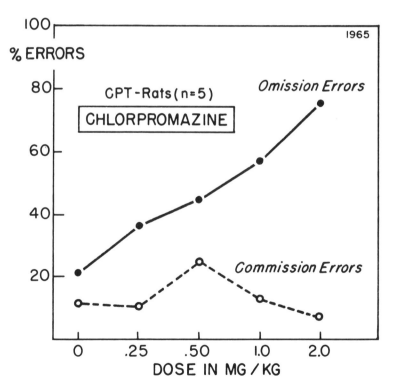

Figure 3.4 Effects of various doses of chlorpromazine on CPT performance in the rat. From Kornetsky and Bain (1965).

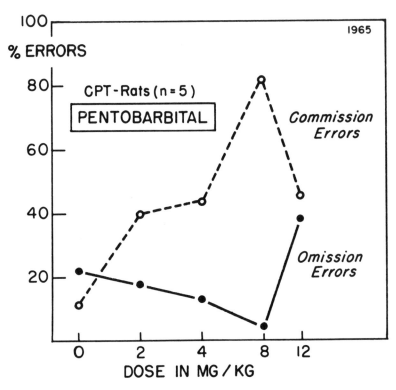

Figure 3.5 Effects of various doses of pentobarbital on CPT performance in the rat. From Kornetsky and Bain (1965).

alcohol-free for at least one week. The normals were from the hospital staff. The three groups were matched for age and level of education. On the DSST the schizophrenics' performance was not significantly different from that of the normals, while the alcoholics performed more poorly than either the normals or the schizophrenics. (It is suggested that this impairment may be related to the changes in cortical functioning frequently seen in chronic alcoholics.) On the CPT the schizophrenics did significantly more poorly than either the normals or the alcoholics. The mean deficit observed was, however, attributable to the performance of only 44% of the schizophrenic subjects tested. (It is suggested in accordance with many diagnostic systems—see, for example, Gromoll (1961)—that we may be dealing with at least two differentiable groups of schizophrenic patients, only one of which is characterized by a dysfunction of the arousal system. In subsequent studies with different samples of hospitalized patients this percentage has held relatively constant.) In clinical studies of patients receiving phenothiazine medication there is marked improvement in the performance on the CPT test, which correlates with clinical observation (Kornetsky, 1972).

In attempting to determine predictors of poor performance on the CPT, we divided a group of chronic schizophrenic patients into two subgroups: (1) those whose performance was indistinguishable from that of normals, and (2) those whose performance was clearly impaired. The performance of these two groups did not differ on the DSST. The patients were assessed by means of two psychiatric rating scales, case histories, and demographic information. Of all the possible predictors of poor performance on the CPT, only a history of mental illness in the family correlated significantly.

Further evidence of an attentional core deficit is given by the experiment of Stammeyer (1961), who matched the performance of schizophrenic subjects with normal subjects on the CPT and found differences between normals and schizophrenics under conditions of sensory overload. When he administered the test with a distracting stimulus (strobe light), he found that the normals' performance improved slightly while that of the schizophrenics became significantly impaired. Using this paradigm, Wohlberg and Kornetsky (1973) compared a group of schizophrenic patients in remission to a group of normals on the CPT under conditions of sensory overload. They found that during the control period there was no significant difference in performance in terms of omission errors; however, there were significant differences during the period when distracting conditions were imposed. The normals showed no change under these conditions, while the schizophrenics became significantly impaired. These were intact schizophrenics in remission, none of them on medication, and many of them holding responsible jobs.

The various experiments described so far demonstrate that some schizophrenic patients perform poorly on a simple test of attention, that chronic phenothiazine administration improves performance on the test, that attention-test performance is vulnerable to the actions of the phenothiazines, that poor performance is related to a history of mental illness in the family, and that the deficit can be uncovered in remitted schizophrenics by means of a sensory overload.

Since all of these experiments, plus the work of others, suggest that the arousal system is involved in the poor performance of some schizophrenics, and since it is postulated that this deficit is a result of central hyperarousal, an animal experiment was designed to model the putative hyperarousal-induced deficit in attention.

The method that was used to cause central activation or arousal was electrical stimulation of the mesencephalic reticular formation while the animal was performing on the animal version of the CPT. If the model is a viable one, then stimulation should impair the animal's performance, and chlorpromazine should attenuate the performance deficit (Kornetsky and Eliasson, 1969). The schematic for this is shown in Figure 3.6. The figure shows an "inverted-U" curve, indicating that, as central activation increases, performance improves up to some undefined maximum. As central activation increases beyond this point, performance declines. This model is not different from the inverted-U curve relating arousal and performance as postulated by Duffy (1957)

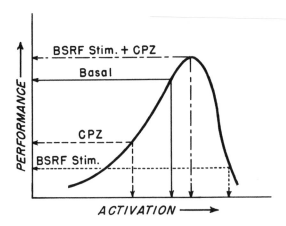

Figure 3.6 An "inverted -U" curve illustrating the postulated relationship between activation and performance. The figure indicates that chlorpromazine reduces activation from basal level, causing impairment in performance, and that reticular stimulation, by moving subjects to the descending leg of the continuum, also impairs performance. When chlorpromazine is combined with stimulation, however, the subject is moved closer to basal activation levels. From Kornetsky and Eliasson (1969). © 1969 by the American Association for the Advancement of Science.

and Malmo (1959), except that the central activation proposed in the present schema does not necessarily imply behavioral arousal. The inverted U as diagrammed indicates that, given the basal level of activation of the animal, chlorpromazine should reduce central arousal and result in impaired performance relative to basal performance (this has already been demonstrated). If, however, central arousal is increased sufficiently, this schema calls for an impairment in performance. And, finally, the inverted U predicts that, if chlorpromazine is administered to the stimulated animal, performance should be significantly better than with either chlorpromazine alone or stimulation alone.

In this experiment an auditory form of the CPT was used, with the critical stimulus a 1200-Hz pure tone and the noncritical stimulus a 1900-Hz tone. Stimulation was delivered by a constant-current stimulator through bipolar electrodes chronically implanted in the mesencephalic reticular formation. Intensities of stimulation were always below those that induce observable behavioral activation. Tones were presented for 1.2 seconds, with the presentation of a tone every 5.0 seconds. The critical stimulus (1200 Hz) was randomly presented an average of once every 6.7 tone presentations. A lever press to the critical stimulus was reinforced by the automatic delivery of a food pellet. A lever press to the noncritical stimulus was an error of commission and postponed the presentation of the next stimulus for 15 seconds. Electrical stimulation during 40% of the interstimulus intervals was randomly presented to the reticular formation. The results of this experiment bore out the prediction: in the three animals studied stimulation alone or chlorpromazine alone impaired performance, but stimulation and chlorpromazine together resulted in a performance level indistinguishable from that of saline alone.

This experiment was replicated using a visual form of the task with two levels of stimulation and two dose levels of chlorpromazine (Eliasson and Kornetsky, 1972). The results replicated those of earlier experiments (see Figure 3.7).

These experiments clearly demonstrate that stimulation of the reticular formation results in impairment on this task and that chlorpromazine in appropriate doses will reverse this effect. However, by itself the experiment does not clearly demonstrate that this is a model for

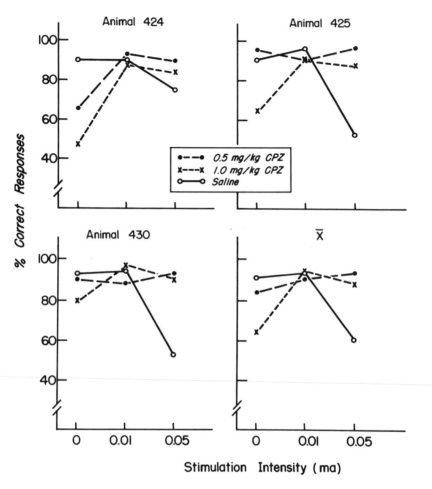

Figure 3.7 The effects of chlorpromazine on percent correct responses as a function of level of stimulation (electrodes in the mesencephalic reticular formation) for each of three animals. Mean percent correct responses are shown on the lower right-hand graph. From Eliasson and Kornetsky (1972).

the impairment on a similar task that is seen in schizophrenic patients. If attention is the critical variable, then stimulating the reticular formation of a rat while it is performing on some other schedule of reinforcement that does not demand sustained attention either should not impair the animal's performance, or, if it does, chlorpromazine should not reverse the effect. Studies by Bain in our laboratory indicate that animals that are trained on either a fixed-ratio or a fixed-interval reinforcement schedule, and that receive reticular stimulation plus chlorpromazine, do not exhibit the behavior seen in the previously described experiments. Figures 3.8 and 3.9 show the results of two such experiments. (Of seven animals used in these two experiments only one animal showed a systematic impairment in performance, as a result of reticular stimulation, that was reversed by chlorpromazine.)

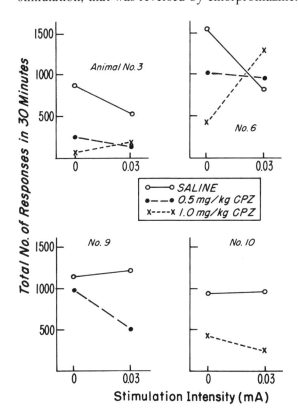

Figure 3.8 Effects of chlorpromazine and reticular stimulation on FR 30 responding.

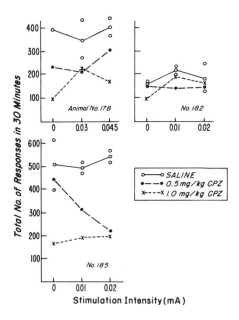

Figure 3.9 Effects of chlorpromazine and reticular stimulation on FI30 seconds responding.

A second question generated by results such as these is whether stimulation of other areas of the brain would give similar results. Unfortunately we have done only a few experiments of this type, but in cases where animals were stimulated accidentally due to inaccurate placement of the electrodes in the central gray or the medial geniculate, or purposeful placement in the raphe nucleus, the results were not similar to those obtained with reticular stimulation. To varying degrees in different animals mixed results were obtained. Either electrical stimulation impaired performance only at stimulation intensities that also produced behavioral activation, or commission errors were increased, or chlorpromazine did not reverse the effects.

A third question that can be asked is: What do nonantipsychotic drugs do in this model? Thus far the only nonantipsychotic drugs tested have been the barbiturates. As shown in Figure 3.5, barbiturates only cause an increase in omission errors when there is also a marked increase in commission errors. If barbiturates are given to an animal concurrently receiving reticular stimulation, omission errors may decrease, but only in the presence of increased commission errors, and in some animals the number of omission errors will increase.

The Role of Norepinephrine

Some attempts have been made to investigate the role of norepinephrine in our attention-deficit model. In one such experiment (Kupferman and Kornetsky, 1971) a stimulating electrode and a push-pull cannula were stereotaxically implanted contralaterally in the reticular formation of the rat. Tritiated norepinephrine was perfused through the cannula for thirty minutes, followed by thirty minutes of perfusion with a label-free solution, before stimulation was started. Electrical stimulation was then given at five-minute intervals, and samples of perfusate were collected each minute. Loss of labeled norepinephrine was an increasing monotonic function of intensity of stimulation. When chlorpromazine was given parenterally prior to the perfusion, the subsequent appearance of norepinephrine in the perfusate collected after stimulation was decreased by a chlorpromazine dose of 1 mg/kg and increased by a dose of 2 mg/kg. These results suggest that disruption of the release and reuptake of norepinephrine may be associated with the stimulation effects and the reversal of chlorpromazine in the behavioral experiments. It is interesting to note that, in almost all behavioral experiments in our laboratories, doses of chlorpromazine have been 1 mg/kg or less.

To further understand the role of norepinephrine in our model, direct application of norepinephrine by means of a push-pull cannula is being studied (Bain and Kornetsky, unpublished data). The animals are implanted with chronic indwelling cannulas, and, after recovery from surgery, are trained on a visual-attention task. For an initial control period the animals are run with only artificial cerebrospinal fluid in the perfusate. At the completion of the predrug period infusion of norepinephrine is begun, and the animals are given approximately 100 trials on the behavioral test. This test period is followed by an additional 25–30 trials with only cerebrospinal fluid in the perfusate. Data obtained thus far clearly indicate that norepinephrine causes an impairment of performance at appropriate concentrations, and at low concentrations it may cause a slight improvement (see Figure 3.10).

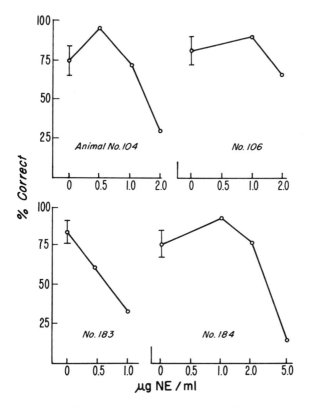

Figure 3.10 Effects of norepinephrine in reticular formation on a visual-attention task.

Summary

As indicated in the first part of this chapter, it is unlikely that an animal model for schizophrenia is possible; however, it is possible that some aspects of the disease state can be modeled.

Of the various behavioral models discussed, some may be no more than bioassays. The CAR seems to fall into this category. The procedure allows for the prediction of antipsychotic activity of drugs in patients, but it tells us very little about the disease process itself.

For a procedure to qualify as a model it need not mimic the disease in its entirety, but it must have some analogous relationship to a significant aspect of the disease that it models. The difficulty is that, given our present state of knowledge, we are not sure what constitutes the relevant or critical aspects of either the disease or the model. Chronic amphetamine abuse produces in man a paranoia-like state and stereotyped behavior. This drug-induced state has been offered as a model of paranoid schizophrenia. In animals amphetamine induces behavioral stereotypies. This drug-induced state is primarily a model of the drug-induced state in man, a model of a model. It *may* also be a model for the human disease. It is possible that the animal stereotypies and the paranoid ideation seen as the result of chronic amphetamine administration in man are parallel phenomena not related in an obligatory fashion, and that only the model paranoia is relevant to the disease. The drug-induced state in the animal may model either a relevant aspect or an irrelevant correlate of the relevant phenomenon in the human model. Considerable scrutiny of these amphetamine models is necessary before their applicability to schizophrenia can be accepted or rejected.

The proposed model of Stein and Wise, despite its logical consistency, is based on the unproven premise that schizophrenia is a disease in which the "reward system" is dysfunctioning. However, the model has generated a continuing series of experiments that should teach us a great deal about the neurochemistry of the "reward system."

The animal model that we have presented is based on the hypothesis that there is a dysfunction of the arousal systems in some schizophrenics. This hypothesis is, in turn, based on extensive experimental evidence that the core deficit in schizophrenic patients is an attentional one. Although the evidence for an attentional deficit in the schizophrenic is clear, the evidence that it is a core deficit, although compelling, is not conclusive. We may simply be modeling some unessential correlate of the disease, and our model may have only a peripheral relationship to the underlying basis of the disease. If this is the case, then the model must, at a minimum, have some relevance in helping to understand the neural system under study.

References

Blum, R. H. 1957. Alpha-rhythm responsiveness in normal, schizophrenic, and brain-damaged persons. *Science* 126:749–750.

Boakes, J., Bradley, P. B., and Candy, J. M. 1972. A neuronal basis for the altering action of (+)-amphetamine. *Br. J. Pharmacol.* 45:391–403.

Bradley, P. B., and Key, B. J. 1968. The effects of drugs on arousal responses produced by electrical stimulation of the reticular formation of the brain. *Electroencephalogr. Clin. Neurophysiol.* 10:560–571.

Brazier, M. A. B., 1972. *The neurophysiological background for anesthesia.* Springfield, Ill.: Charles C Thomas.

Crow, T. J. 1972. Catecholamine-containing neurones and electrical self-stimulation: 1. A review of some data. *Psychol. Med.* 2:414–421.

Crow, T. J. 1973. Catecholamine-containing neurones and electrical self-stimulation: 2. A theoretical interpretation and some psychiatric implications. *Psychol. Med.* 3:66–73.

Duffy, E. 1957. The psychological significance of a concept of "arousal" or "activation." *Psychol. Rev.* 64:265.

Eliasson, M., and Kornetsky, C. 1972. Interaction effects of chlorpromazine and reticular stimulation on visual attention behavior in rats. *Psychon. Sci.* 26:261–262.

Ellinwood, E. H., Sudilovsky, A., and Nelson, L. 1972. Behavioral analysis of chronic amphetamine intoxication. *Biol. Psychiatry* 4:3.

Fedio, P., Mirsky, A. F., Smith, W. J., and Parry, D. 1961. Reaction time and EEG activation in normal and schizophrenic subjects. *Electroencephalogr. Clin. Neurophysiol.* 13:923–926.

Feldstein, A. 1970. Biochemical aspects of schizophrenia and antipsychotic drugs. In A. DiMascio and R. Schader, eds., *Clinical handbook of psychopharmacology.* New York: Science House.

Gerard, R. W., 1956. *Neuropharmacology: Transactions of the second conference.* New York: Josiah Macy, Jr. Foundation.

Griffith, J. D., Cavanaugh, J., Held, J., and Oates, J. A. 1972. Dextroamphetamine— Evaluation of psychotomimetic properties in man. *Arch. Gen. Psychiatry* 26:97–100.

Gromoll, H. G. 1961. The process-reactive dimension of schizophrenia in relation to cortical activation and arousal. Ph.D. dissertation, University of Illinois, Urbana, Illinois.

Hill, D. 1957. Electroencephalogram in schizophrenia. In D. Richter, ed., *Schizophrenia: Somatic Aspects.* Oxford: Pergamon.

Hollister, L. E. 1968. *Chemical psychoses: LSD and related drugs.* Springfield, Ill.: Charles C Thomas.

Kornetsky, C. 1972. The use of a simple test of attention as a measure of drug effects in schizophrenic patients. *Psychopharmacologia* 24:99–106.

Kornetsky, C., and Bain, G. 1965. The effects of chlorpromazine and pentobarbital on sustained attention in the rat. *Psychopharmacologia* 8:277.

Kornetsky, C., and Eliasson, M. 1969. Reticular stimulation and chlorpromazine: An animal model for schizophrenic overarousal. *Science* 165:1273–1274.

Kornetsky, C., and Mirsky, A. F. 1966. On certain psychopharmacologic and physiological differences between schizophrenics and normal persons. *Psychopharmacologia* 14:309–318.

Kupferman, A., and Kornetsky, C. 1971. The effect of chlorpromazine on the release of 7-H^3-norepinephrine by electrical stimulation of the rat mesencephalic reticular formation. *The Pharmacologist* 13:217 (abstract).

Machiyama, Y., Utena, H., and Kikuchi, M. 1970. Behavioral disorders in Japanese monkeys produced by the long-term administration of methamphetamine. *Proc. Jap. Acad.* 7:738–743.

Malmo, R. A. 1959. Activation: a neuropsychological dimension. *Psychol. Rev.* 66:367.

Mirsky, A. F., and Kornetsky, C. 1964. On the dissimilar effects of drugs on the digit symbol substitution and continuous performance tests. *Psychopharmacologia* 5:161.

Olds, J., and Milner, P. 1954. Positive reinforcement produced by electrical stimulation of septal area and other regions of rat brain. *J. Comp. Physiol. Psychol.* 47:419–427.

Orzack, M., and Kornetsky, C. 1966. Attention dysfunction in chronic schizophrenia. *Arch. Gen. Psychiatry* 14:323–326.

Rosvold, H. E., Mirsky, A. F., Sarason, L., Bransome, E. D., and Beck, L. H. 1965. A continuous performance test of brain damage. *J. Consult. Psychol.* 114:1004.

Shakow, D. 1962. Segmental set. *Arch. Gen. Psychiatry* 6:1–17.

Smythies, J. R., ed. 1970. *The mode of action of psychotomimetic drugs.* (*Neurosci. Res. Program Bull.,* vol. 8, no. 1.)

Snyder, S. H. 1973. Amphetamine psychosis: A model schizophrenia mediated by catecholamines. *Am. J. Psychiatry* 130:61–67.

Stammeyer, E. C. 1961. *The effects of distraction on performance in schizophrenic, psychoneurotic, and normal individuals.* Washington: The Catholic University of America Press.

Stein, L. 1964. Reciprocal action of reward and punishment mechanisms. In R. G. Heath, ed., *Role of pleasure in behavior.* New York: Hoeber.

Stein, L., and Wise, C. D. 1971. Possible etiology of schizophrenia: Progressive damage of the noradrenergic reward mechanism by endogenous 6-hydroxydopamine. *Science* 171:1032.

Venables, P. H. 1964. Input dysfunction in schizophrenia. In B. A. Maher, ed. *Progress in experimental personality research.* New York: Academic Press.

Venables, P. H., and Wing, J. K. 1962. Level of arousal and the subclassification of schizophrenia. *Arch. Gen. Psychiatry* 7:114–119.

Wohlberg, G. W., and Kornetsky, C. 1973. Sustained attention in remitted schizophrenics. *Arch. Gen. Psychiatry* 28:533–537.

Wyatt, R. J., Saavedra, J. M., and Axelrod, J. 1973. A dimethyltryptamine-forming enzyme in human blood. *Am. J. Psychiatry* 130:7.

4

Biological Models in the Study of False Neurochemical Synaptic Transmitters

Ross J. Baldessarini and Josef E. Fischer

In the present chapter the process of "modeling" will be utilized at several levels of biological complexity. In our studies of a novel means by which disordered function can occur at synapses in the central nervous system, the process of model construction was applied at the levels of the subcellular organelle, of tissue and organ function, and of the whole animal as we investigated the role of relatively inactive and thus "false" neurotransmitters in hepatic encephalopathy. This topic of study is itself perhaps a "model" (i.e., an illustrative example) for the application of the concept of false transmission to a broader range of more subtle pharmacological and neuropsychiatric problems. The term "model" in the present context simply means an experimental compromise in that a simple experimental system is used to represent a more complex and less readily accessible system: the animal to represent the patient, the tissue slice to represent the intact living brain, the isolated nerve ending to represent the intact synapse.

Disordered Amine Metabolism and Neuropsychiatric Illness

There has been a great deal of interest in recent years in the function of biogenic amines as probable neurochemical transmitters at synapses in the brain; it has repeatedly been suggested that disorders of amine metabolism occur in the affective disorders (Baldessarini, 1975) and the schizophrenias (Kety and Matthysse, 1972). There is considerable evidence that many of the drugs used in psychiatry have important interactions with synaptic transmission in the brain, particularly in systems that utilize catecholamines and indoleamines as their

R. J. Baldessarini, Department of Psychiatry, and J. E. Fischer, Department of Surgery, Massachusetts General Hospital, Boston, MA, 02114. This work was supported by the following U.S. Public Health Service Research Grants: NIMH Grant MH-16674, General Research Support Grant FR-05486, and NAIMD Grant RO1-AM 15347 PHRA. RJB is recipient of NIMH Research Scientist Career Development Award KO2-MH-74370.

neurotransmitters. These systems have important regulatory functions in relation to the autonomic nervous system and may also subserve such higher functions as arousal and affect (Baldessarini, 1972). Much of the speculation concerning the possible relationship of disordered amine metabolism to mental illness derives from the inference that, if drugs which have beneficial clinical effects also have important interactions with aminergic synapses in the brain, then a pathophysiological basis of the illness may include a disorder of the function of synapses. Of course, to argue on the basis of drug effects is to risk the construction of hypotheses on logically shaky ground, but, unfortunately, more direct evidence of spontaneously abnormal synaptic metabolism in idiopathic mental illness is for the most part either lacking or, at best, inconsistent and unconvincing. Thus it is possible that the hypothetical connection between mental illness and disordered synaptic function is more apparent than real.

A more satisfying way to relate synaptic dysfunction to neuro-psychiatric illness is to have clinical metabolic data to support the pharmacological and neurochemical work done in the laboratory with animals or with their tissues. This has been the approach we have adopted in our studies. The price of the increased scientific satisfaction is that one is forced to study more obviously "metabolic" diseases, such as the encephalopathy associated with liver failure in the present instance, and to risk "irrelevance" with respect to the idiopathic psychoses. However, since so little is known about the normal and pathologic functions of amines and amino acids in the brain, such studies may not be altogether trivial and irrelevant to clinical issues in neuropsychiatry.

The Concept of False Transmission

The concept of "false" neurochemical transmitters evolved in the 1960s as a means of explaining certain pharmacological observations concerning the peripheral sympathetic nervous system (Kopin, 1968). Thus, for example, the hypotensive effects of α-methylated analogues of *m*-tyrosine and dihydroxyphenylalanine (DOPA) were believed to result at least partly from their conversion by decarboxylation and β-hydroxylation to relatively inactive structural analogues of norepinephrine, the normal sympathetic transmitter, in the periphery, as well as to analogues of either norepinephrine or dopamine in the brain. It has also been hypothesized that the hypotensive effects and diminution of the pain (angina pectoris) associated with coronary artery disease which sometimes result from the chronic treatment of patients with inhibitors of the enzyme monoamine oxidase (MAO)—a major means of inactivating biologically active amines—might also be due to the accumulation in nerve endings of amine products that are usually destroyed by MAO. From studies of the sympathetic nervous system it appears that the structural requirements of a false transmitter include a phenyl-ethyl-amine configuration. Furthermore at least one phenolic hydroxyl group is required, and, in order for such molecules to be stored in nerve endings and to be released by neural activity, it is believed that they should have another hydroxyl group on the benzene ring or on the β carbon of the side chain (Kopin, 1968; Fischer et al., 1965). Such compounds are relatively weak directly acting sympathomimetic amines if they also lack a second hydroxyl group on the benzene ring or if they have a methyl group on the α carbon of the side chain.

Such phenomena may also occur in the central nervous system (CNS) since there is a rapidly growing body of evidence to suggest that aromatic amines may serve as physiological neurotransmitters there. The evidence is perhaps most compelling for the catecholamines norepinephrine and dopamine, although there is also quite good evidence for serotonin and for a variety of excitatory and inhibitory amino acids (Phyllis, 1970; Baldessarini and Karobath, 1973). Since little is known about the metabolism of other aromatic amines in the CNS, and even less is known about their metabolism in neuropsychiatric patients, we have been studying basic aspects of the metabolism of such amines. More specifically, we have studied hepatic failure as an example of a condition in which abnormal metabolism of amines might occur (Fischer and Baldessarini, 1971). Hepatic failure is an attractive model because it includes clinical signs of altered function of peripheral adrenergic transmission in addition to neuropsychiatric signs of CNS dysfunction.

Hepatic Failure as a Model of False Transmission
In hepatic failure precursors of possible false transmitters are readily available. They include the aromatic amino acids provided by protein and their corresponding amines produced in the gut by the action of

bacterial amino-acid decarboxylases. Normally, exogenous aromatic amines are largely catabolized by MAO, notably in the liver, and so cleared from the portal blood. When hepatic function is impaired and blood is shunted around the liver, precursors can flood the nervous system. Aromatic amino acids can be locally decarboxylated in brain tissue to their corresponding amines by a relatively nonspecific decarboxylase. Certain amines might then be locally β-hydroxylated by another relatively nonspecific oxidizing enzyme localized in nerve endings and so might replace normal adrenergic transmitters. The metabolic pathways pertinent to this discussion are summarized in Figure 4.1.

Certain cardiovascular and renal complications, including the high-cardiac-output, low-peripheral-vascular-resistance state and the uremia ("hepatorenal syndrome") which may occur in severe liver failure, could result from the replacement of norepinephrine by weakly sympathomimetic amines, resulting in loss of arteriolar tone, opening of peripheral vascular shunts, perfusion of nonessential areas, and shunting of blood away from the kidneys. Similarly asterixis or flapping tremor, a sign of extrapyramidal dysfunction, might result from a displacement of transmitters in the basal ganglia, for example, where dopamine is a physiological transmitter; dopamine is also deficient in the brains of patients with paralysis agitans (Parkinson's disease). Disturbances of consciousness in hepatic coma might be due to displacement of various transmitter substances from widely distributed central neuronal systems since there is evidence of an altered metabolism of biogenic amines in the altered states of consciousness induced by drugs or by lesions of the brainstem (Baldessarini, 1972).

A false-transmitter hypothesis for hepatic coma is consistent with certain clinical features of this condition (Fischer, 1975). Thus shunting of portal blood around the liver and loss of hepatic function would diminish both the utilization of amino acids and the catabolism of amines present in portal blood. Ammonia and other nitrogenous products would accumulate in the systemic circulation, but, since the clinical condition would depend on the accumulation of amines in nerve endings, serum levels of ammonia would not necessarily reflect tissue levels of amines, particularly in the brain, and do not correlate closely

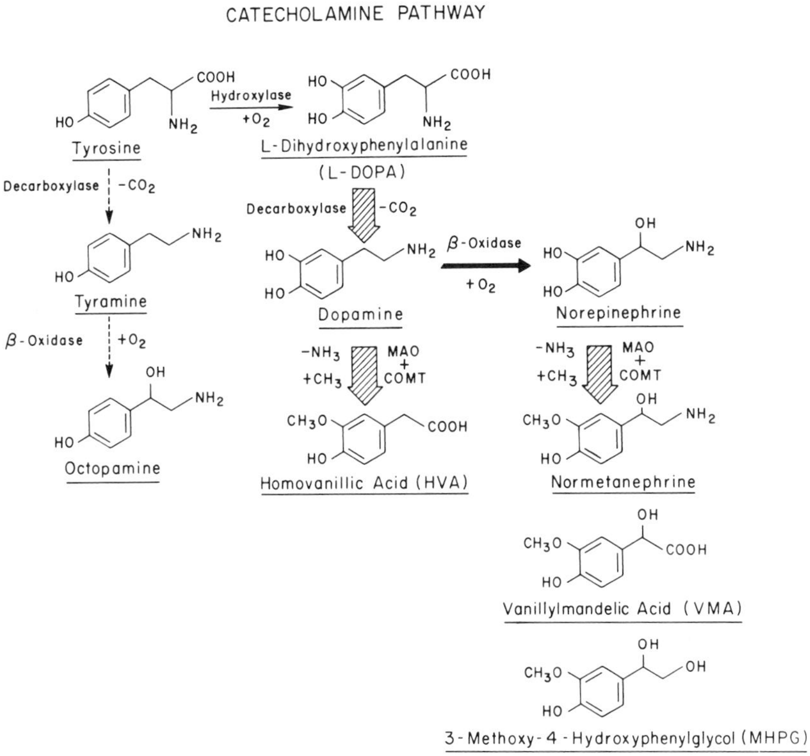

CATECHOLAMINE PATHWAY

Figure 4.1 Metabolic pathway of the catecholamines and related phenylethylamines in the mammalian central nervous system.

with the neuropsychiatric status of patients with hepatic failure.

Since amines can be produced by the action of bacteria on the amino acids presented by dietary protein or bleeding into the gut (a common complication of hepatic failure), a greater availability of protein should increase the opportunity to accumulate amines, and does in fact make hepatic encephalopathy worse in man and in animals. Conversely, withholding protein or "sterilizing" the gut with poorly absorbed antibiotics would be expected to reduce the formation of amines, and these steps often bring about clinical improvement of the patient's mental status (Fischer and Baldessarini, 1972; Fischer et al., 1972; Fischer, 1975). In the dog brain increased levels of aromatic amino acids have been reported to occur in hepatic coma. However, on the whole, very little attention has been given to the assay of amine concentrations in animals or patients with hepatic encephalopathy, although high circulating levels of β-phenethylamine have been reported to occur in patients.

Experimental Models of Hepatic Failure

In our initial studies of the potential of aromatic amines to interfere with the storage and retention of physiologically important catecholamines in nerve terminals of the brain, attempts were made to develop models of the proposed clinical situation. Thus we administered aromatic amines to laboratory rats and chemically assayed the concentrations of catecholamines in their tissues. When large doses of β-phenethylamine were given to rats, norepinephrine levels were markedly decreased in their hearts and brains, while tyramine, a more polar phenolic amine which apparently passes the blood-brain diffusion barrier less easily, depleted stores of the neurotransmitter in peripheral tissues only. Furthermore only with phenethylamine did we note the occurrence of marked behavioral effects, including the bizarre posturing and compulsive gnawing behaviors which have been reported to occur after treatment with large doses of amphetamines and which may be mediated by increased transmission in the dopamine-containing neurons of the basal ganglia (Randrup and Munkvad, 1970).

In another attempt to model the proposed metabolic abnormalities of hepatic failure we administered large doses of aromatic amino acids to rats in which either the hepatic circulation was altered surgically or the hepatic function was altered pharmacologically, and we then assayed tissue levels of several aromatic amines that are normally present in only very low concentrations. Compromise of hepatic function was produced by pretreating the animals with an inhibitor of MAO, or by surgically diverting the portal blood flow away from the liver directly into the systemic circulation at the vena cava, while leaving hepatic MAO activity unchanged. In these experiments we found striking accumulations of phenylethanolamine as well as of its phenolic derivative, octopamine (see Figure 4.1), in peripheral sympathetically innervated tissues as well as in the brain (Table 4.1).

In Vitro Experimental Models
We then decided to pursue the study of several representative aromatic amines in brain tissue more closely in order to find out whether they can act as substitute neurotransmitters. In the past the biochemical physiology of nerve terminals in the peripheral nervous system has been studied with isolated organs, such as the heart or the spleen, perfused through an arterial cannula with physiological solutions collected as a venous effluent. Nerves to the tissue are isolated and stimulated, and the resulting changes in levels of metabolites in the perfusate can be correlated with the effects of stimulation of the nerves.

Unfortunately similar approaches to the study of nerve terminals have not been possible in the CNS because of its anatomical complexity and

Table 4.1
The accumulation of octopamine in rat tissue (ng/organ $\pm$ S.E.M.)

	Octopamine in heart	Octopamine in brain
Control	78 $\pm$ 3	4 $\pm$ 1
Pargyline administered	104 $\pm$ 9*	34 $\pm$ 4*
Pargyline + phenylalanine administered	240 $\pm$ 20*	59 $\pm$ 8*
Portacaval shunt	112 $\pm$ 18*	17 $\pm$ 4*

* $p < 0.01$ by t-test; N $\geq$ 6.
Rats were given pargyline (20 mg/kg) intraperitoneally or oral L-phenylalanine (250 mg/kg) daily for four days and were killed two hours after the last dose. Controls with either saline injections or sham operations were not different and are pooled. Pargyline is a potent MAO inhibitor.

inaccessibility. Nevertheless certain approaches are possible, including experiments that might be considered "models" of presently unattainable perfusions of specific populations of isolated central nerve terminals. For example, one can keep slices of brain tissue more or less "alive" in oxygenated physiological solutions in vitro and thus study many aspects of their metabolism, including the uptake, synthesis, and storage of amino acids and amines. One can also stimulate such tissues with electrical fields or increased concentrations of potassium ion in the incubation medium by superfusing the brain slices in glass or plastic chambers, and this preparation can be used as a model with which to study the release of putative neurotransmitters.

Furthermore it is now possible to homogenize brain tissue under conditions that permit the region of the nerve terminal to be "pinched off" in a more or less intact form. Such subcellular structures can then be recovered highly selectively by ultracentrifugation techniques. They tend to reseal into micron-sized spheres, enclosed by the cell membrane of the presynaptic region of the nerve terminal (often with some portions of the postsynaptic membrane still attached), and contain cytoplasm, mitochondria, and granules or vesicles believed to represent presynaptic storage sites for various neurotransmitters. These subcellular fragments are commonly called "synaptosomes" (Figure 4.2). They retain a remarkable variety of metabolic functions believed to be associated with intact nerve terminals, including the ability to respire, to synthesize adenosine triphosphate, to transport amino acids, to synthesize protein, and to synthesize, take up, store, and perhaps even release amine neurotransmitters (Baldessarini and Karobath, 1973) (see Figure 4.3). The attraction of such simplified tissue preparations is that they allow biochemical and pharmacological experiments to be performed under carefully controlled conditions. The obvious disadvantage is that they represent a serious compromise with respect to the physiological realities of the intact nervous system.

In these experiments we have found that several radioactive phenyl-ethylamine derivatives are taken up and retained by slices of brain and by isolated nerve endings (synaptosomes). This storage increases with the degree of hydroxylation of the amines in the ascending order β-phen-ethylamine $<$ tyramine $<$ octopamine $<$ norepinephrine. The uptake or transport of the amines is saturable with increasing concentrations of the

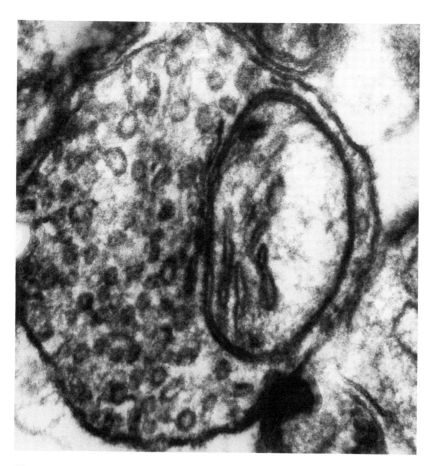

Figure 4.2 Electron micrograph of a typical "pinched-off" nerve ending (synaptosome) prepared from rat cerebral cortex by subcellular fractionation (diameter is 1–2 μm).

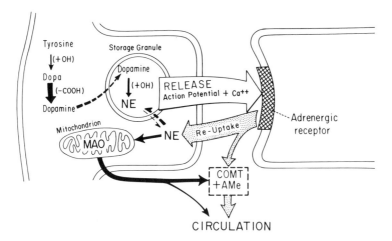

PRESYNAPTIC NEURON   **POSTSYNAPTIC NEURON**

Figure 4.3 Scheme or summarizing "model" of the important steps believed to occur at a typical adrenergic nerve terminal. Synthesis occurs from phenylalanine or tyrosine by the action of tyrosine hydroxylase, a rate-limiting step. DOPA is converted to the amine by a relatively nonspecific aromatic amino acid decarboxylase, and dopamine is then β-hydroxylated by another relatively nonspecific enzyme, phenylethylamine β-hydroxylase, to norepinephrine. The transmitter is stored in presynaptic vesicles. Release occurs upon intrusion of the action potential and requires calcium ion. A poorly understood postsynaptic action then occurs between the amine and its "receptor." The sequence is terminated mainly by a vigorous and specific reuptake process which also helps to conserve the neurotransmitter (and permits selective labeling of the nerve terminal with radioactive amine). In addition enzymatic processes exist to scavenge any remaining amine not reaccumulated, including monoamine oxidase (MAO) and catechol-O-methyl-transferase (COMT), which requires S-adenosyl-methionine (AMe) as methyl donor.

substrate, with transport constants (substrate concentrations at half-maximal uptake velocity, analogous to "K_m"—the Michaelis constant—in enzymology) on the order of 0.1 to 10.0 μM (Figure 4.4). Similar "high-affinity" transport processes (low transport constants) occur with nearly every amine or amino acid suspected of being a neurotransmitter in the central nervous system (with the probable exception of acetylcholine) (Baldessarini and Karobath, 1973).

The uptake of the hydroxylated amines tyramine, octopamine, and norepinephrine is much more vigorous in striatal tissue (caudate nucleus and putamen) than in cerebral cortical tissue, and their uptake is inhibited by reduced temperature, by lack of glucose, by metabolic poisons, and by drugs that are known to inhibit the uptake of the catecholamines (desmethylimipramine, cocaine, and ouabain). The uptake of norepinephrine and octopamine appears to require sodium ions. Pretreatment of rats with reserpine (which blocks intraneuronal storage of amines) or with 6-hydroxydopamine (which itself is a kind of false transmitter and selectively destroys catecholamine-containing nerve endings) decreases the ability of brain tissues to take up and store norepinephrine or octopamine.

Previously accumulated labeled phenylethylamines migrate in sucrose density gradients with a peak of radioactivity corresponding to an equilibrium position of catecholamine-containing nerve endings (Figure 4.5). The magnitude of the retention of labeled amines in this synaptosomal peak decreases in the order norepinephrine $>$octopamine $>$tyramine. The accumulated amines are released by the sonic, osmotic, and thermal stresses that disrupt neuronal membranes. During superfusion, tyramine and metaraminol (α-methyl-β-hydroxy-m-tyramine) displace [^{3}H]norepinephrine from binding sites in brain slices (Figure 4.6). In general the presence of a β-hydroxyl group appears to protect amines from destruction by MAO in cerebral cortical tissue, presumably by virtue of uptake into presynaptic vesicles.

When the release of aromatic amines was studied (Baldessarini and Vogt, 1972), we found that the radioactive β-hydroxylated phenylethylamines octopamine and metaraminol, as well as norepinephrine, are released by either electrical stimulation or increased concentrations of K^+ from preparations of rat brain containing mainly cerebral cortex (Figure 4.7). In contrast amphetamine and tyramine are

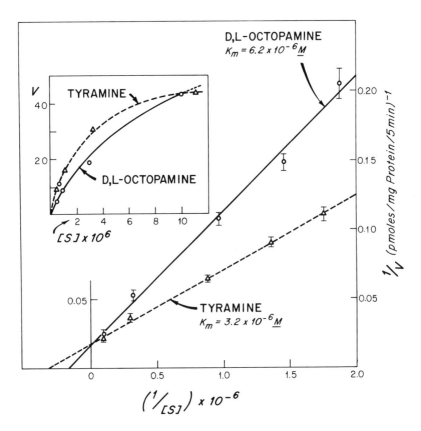

Figure 4.4 Uptake of aromatic amines by isolated nerve endings. Synaptosomes prepared from rat brain were incubated with increasing concentrations of labeled tyramine and octopamine and then transport was found to follow saturable kinetics with a very low transport constant ("high-affinity" uptake) (N = 6).

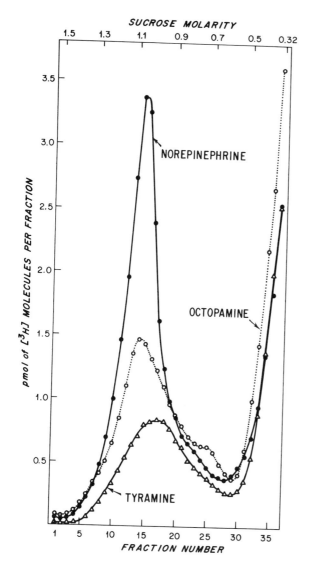

Figure 4.5 Subcellular distribution of ³H following incubation of labeled amines with minces of rat brain. Tissues were homogenized in isotonic sucrose and centrifuged at 100,000 × g on continuous sucrose density gradients. Data are means of three experiments.

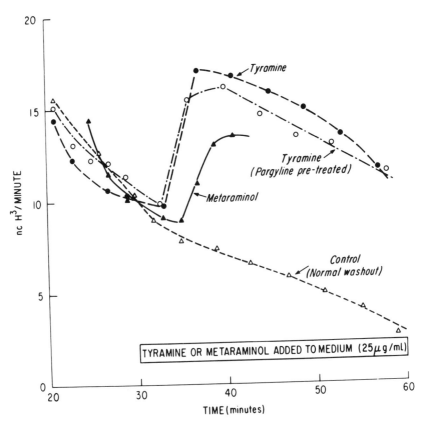

Figure 4.6 Displacement of [³H]norepinephrine from slices of rat brain by amines added to a physiological superfusing medium. Slices were preincubated with [³H]norepinephrine, washed, and superfused in glass chambers. The ³H in the effluent was counted.

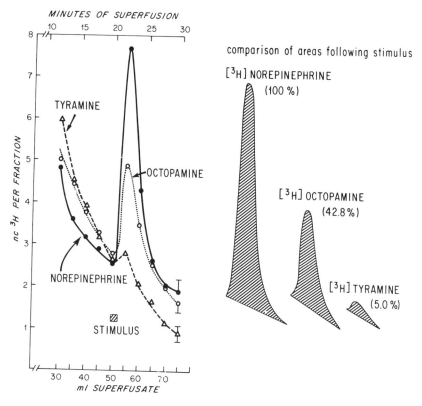

Figure 4.7 Release of [³H]-labeled amines from slices of rat brain pretreated with a MAO inhibitor. Tissues containing mainly cerebral cortex were preincubated with each amine, washed, and superfused in glass chambers with a physiological medium. An alternating electrical-field stimulus was applied for 60 seconds. Data are means of ten experiments ± S.E.M. (vertical lines).

poorly released from cortex, and the release of urea or leucine is barely perceptible. The addition of unlabeled norepinephrine to an incubating medium leads to displacement of previously bound [³H]-labeled octopamine or metaraminol from a preparation of isolated nerve endings. Pretreatment of rats with intracisternal 6-hydroxydopamine markedly decreases the ability of slices of cerebral cortex to release [³H]norepinephrine or [³H]octopamine. When the release of amines was studied regionally, we found that the release of [³H]norepinephrine appears to parallel the endogenous distribution of this amine. Exogenous dopamine (not β-hydroxylated) or octopamine (not a catechol) are released well from caudate nucleus, hypothalamus, or cerebral cortex. The behavior of the tyramines (para- or meta-hydroxylated) is very different in that they are released quite well from the caudate nucleus, somewhat less well from the hypothalamus, but poorly from minces of cerebral cortex (Figure 4.8).

In summary these results strongly suggest (1) that a variety of amines can interfere with the retention of those amines that are probably physiological transmitters and (2) that hydroxylated amines can be taken up and stored in nerve endings of the brain. If the compounds are β-hydroxylated (e.g., octopamine and metaraminol), they apparently can be stored in and released from nerve endings in which the normal transmitter is either β-hydroxylated (norepinephrine) or not (dopamine), while non-β-hydroxylated analogues (e.g., p- or m-tyramine) are more poorly stored in the former nerve endings but are apparently relatively successfully stored in and released from terminals in which the normal transmitter is not β-hydroxylated (e.g., dopamine in the neostriatum).

In Vivo Experimental Models

In other experiments an animal model of acute hepatic coma was produced in rats by ligation of the hepatic artery 24 hours after end-to-side portacaval venous shunts were constructed. If the animals were maintained with glucose infusions, they survived the second procedure for 8–10 hours, with gradually increasing somnolence and then coma. Control animals were subjected only to sham operations and similar infusions. Animals in coma had decreased levels of norepinephrine in their brains and hearts and small decreases of dopamine in their brains (Table 4.2). When β-hydroxylated

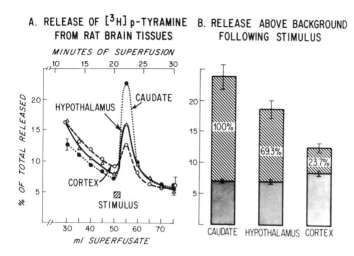

Figure 4.8 Release of [³H]*p*-tyramine from minces of rat brain prepared from specific regions. A: The tissues were incubated with [³H]tyramine following treatment with a MAO inhibitor, washed, superfused, and stimulated as for Figure 4.7. B: Release was compared by bar graphs representing the area under peaked curves following stimulation. The striped areas are compared as percentages of the maximum release (from striatal tissue) above spontaneous efflux (shaded lower portions of bars). Data are presented as percentages of total ³H released during the 20 minutes of superfusion.

Table 4.2
Catecholamines in experimental hepatic coma (ng/g ± S.E.M.)

	Norepinephrine	Dopamine
Brain		
Control	394 ± 32	811 ± 64
Coma	180 ± 17*	725 ± 96
	(46%)	(89%)
Heart		
Control	699 ± 29	
Coma	573 ± 94	
	(82%)	

* p < 0.01 by t-test; N ≥ 10.
Endogenous amines were measured in the tissues of rats in hepatic coma following portacaval anastomosis and ligation of the hepatic artery. Controls had sham operations.

phenylethylamines were assayed, increased amounts of octopamine were found in heart and brain, with more striking increases as the coma deepened (Table 4.3). Similar results were obtained in assays of phenylethanolamine, and we also observed consistent increases in concentrations of serotonin. These increases may reflect decreased destruction of amines in the toxic animals or the greater availability of precursors in the systemic circulation. Furthermore increased urinary excretion of octopamine with increased severity of the neuropsychiatric dysfunction of patients in hepatic failure was also observed (Table 4.4), helping to support the proposal that the surgically prepared animal model provides at least partly valid comparisons with clinically observed cases of hepatic failure.

One limitation of this particular animal model is that the rat is relatively resistant to the production of coma by less catastrophic surgical interventions, such as portacaval venous anastomosis alone. Since the ligation of the hepatic artery leads to an acute insult to the liver and a variety of serious metabolic derangements, coma produced in this way may not really provide a fair comparison to the clinical situation.

On the one hand rats have the advantage that they are inexpensive and

Table 4.3
Octopamine levels in moderate or severe experimental acute hepatic coma
(ng/organ ± S.E.M.)

	Brain	Heart
Control	6 ± 1	73 ± 12
"Somnolent"	12 ± 2*	100 ± 22*
Severe coma	24 ± 4*	179 ± 26*

* $p < 0.01$ by t-test; $N \geq 7$.
Coma was produced by a two-stage interruption of the hepatic blood supply. Controls had sham operations.

Table 4.4
Twenty-four hour urinary octopamine excretion in patients with hepatic failure who had flapping tremor (asterixis) and minimal disorientation or frank hepatic coma
(μg/24 hr ± S.E.M.)

	N	Octopamine
Control	11	1.1 ± 0.3
Asterixis	5	2.6 ± 0.5 ($p < 0.02$)
Coma	6	5.0 ± 1.2 ($p < 0.01$)

can be sacrificed in large numbers for a broad range of biochemical studies of brain tissue. On the other hand it is well known that larger animals, classically the dog, with a portacaval anastomosis (Eck's fistula) can easily be intoxicated with protein or amino-acid feedings. We have found this to be true in dogs and monkeys with such surgical diversions of the portal blood away from the liver. Thus it is possible to produce chronic and also reversible states of confusion and coma in such large animals and to test a variety of potentially therapeutic interventions in these model situations. The disadvantages are that the large animals are expensive to prepare and to support and do not readily lend themselves to biochemical analyses of brain tissue. The latter disadvantage may be offset by the availability of urine, blood, and cerebrospinal fluid for chemical analysis in these large animals.

Other Possible False Transmitters: Serotonin and Glutamine
Thus far we have emphasized the possible association between increased accumulations of phenylethylamine compounds in hepatic failure and the pathophysiology of the neurological features of the condition. This emphasis may very well be shortsighted, and it is very strongly biased by the availability of a substantial literature on aromatic amines as false neurotransmitters in the peripheral sympathetic nervous system (Kopin, 1968), a model that has strongly influenced our thinking about the brain. However, it is highly probable that a variety of other amines and amino acids also serve as normal neurotransmitters or "modulators" of synaptic function in the brain (Baldessarini and Karobath, 1973), and it is equally likely that hepatic failure is associated with a variety of metabolic anomalies (Fischer, 1975).

One of the amines that is likely to act as a physiological transmitter in certain central neurons, serotonin (5-hydroxytryptamine), has several other properties that make it interesting in the present context (Baldessarini and Fischer, 1973). These include the possibility that it may accumulate in neurons in which it is not normally located, including adrenergic neurons in the periphery and in the brain. Evidence for this phenomenon includes the observation that intra-arterially injected serotonin can release epinephrine from the dog adrenal gland. It is also known that serotonin derived from its precursor amino acids can displace catecholamines from brain slices in vitro, and that it can release dopamine in vivo, as indicated by a rise in the cerebrospinal-fluid concentrations of its major metabolite, homovanillic acid. It is also known that patients in liver failure are intolerant to tryptophan, the precursor of the indoleamines—intolerant both clinically (increased mental confusion) and biochemically (less able to clear tryptophan from the blood). One of the interesting aspects of the synthesis of the indoleamines is that the enzyme which 5-hydroxylates tryptophan, while rate-limiting in the synthesis of serotonin, is normally not saturated with substrate at physiological levels of tryptophan. Thus it is possible to "push" the synthesis of serotonin by increasing tryptophan levels. We have found that a portacaval venous anastomosis leads to markedly increased levels of tryptophan, serotonin, and the main metabolite of serotonin, 5-hydroxyindoleacetic acid, in the rat brain (Table 4.5). Since increased tryptophan is available in the systemic circulation of patients in liver failure, it is conceivable that increased accumulations of indoleamines in anomalous locations, for example in central catecholamine nerve terminals, might thus represent another false-transmitter mechanism.

Although it has not previously been suggested, it is also possible that amino acids acting as neurotransmitters in the brain might also be influenced by false-transmitter mechanisms. One possibility pertinent to hepatic encephalopathy is that glutamine, a neurophysiologically

Table 4.5
Effects of the surgical diversion of portal blood flow and L-DOPA on indole metabolism in the rat brain

	Brain Concentration (μg/g $\pm$ S.E.M.)		
	Tryptophan	Serotonin	5-Hydroxyindoleacetic acid
Control	4.9 $\pm$ 0.4 (100%)	0.48 $\pm$ 0.02 (100%)	0.37 $\pm$ 0.02 (100%)
Shunted	13.3 $\pm$ 2.0 (273%)	0.71 $\pm$ 0.04 (149%)	0.68 $\pm$ 0.06 (186%)
Shunted + L-DOPA administered	18.6 $\pm$ 1.1 (379%)	0.33 $\pm$ 0.06 (70%)	0.92 $\pm$ 0.04 (251%)

Portacaval anastomosis ("shunted") or sham operations were done in rats, which were sacrificed two months later, when stable. Some rats were also given 100 mg/kg of L-DOPA or its vehicle by nasogastric tube one hour prior to sacrifice. All increases in the untreated shunted rats are significant ($p < 0.001$) when compared to controls by t-test; average $N = 8$.

inactive substance when applied to nerve cells by microiontophoresis, is one of the few metabolites that accumulate in the cerebrospinal fluid in quite consistent correlation with the clinical status of patients. Since glutamine is physiologically inactive and is a close structural analogue of glutamic acid, which is thought to be an excitatory neurotransmitter, it is a good candidate as a false transmitter. It had been thought that glutamine represents an inactive end product of ammonia fixation (two moles of ammonia are used in the conversion of α-oxoglutarate to glutamine). This pathway may represent a process of detoxification under conditions of ammonia accumulation, as in liver disease. However, it was also believed that this pathway could put a "drain" on the Krebs cycle, leading to depletion of α-oxoglutarate and to eventual decreases of adenosine triphosphate (ATP) by this mechanism and also by the utilization of ATP in the synthesis of glutamine from glutamic acid. Recent experiments with experimental ammonia intoxication in the rat have shown that the predicted depletion of Krebs-cycle metabolites and of phosphorylated nucleotides does not occur.

One other finding suggesting that an alternative evaluation of the role of glutamine is necessary is that blockade of the synthesis of glutamine in animals by experimentally induced ammonia intoxication can lead to an improvement in their neurological status, even though ammonia levels become even higher than they are when the glutamine-synthetase step is active (Warren and Schenker, 1964). This finding also tends to diminish the likelihood that ammonia itself is a uniquely important toxin in hepatic encephalopathy.

We have recently found that glutamine can be transported into isolated nerve endings and that this uptake is competitive with the transport of glutamic acid, suggesting that a similar membrane "carrier" mechanism is utilized by both amino acids. We also find that labeled glutamine, unlike many other amino acids, can be released from brain slices by either depolarization with electrical fields or increased concentrations of K^+ (Figure 4.9). These findings support the suggestion that glutamine—an inactive substance—might accumulate in central nerve terminals and might thus by competition decrease the action of other amino acids that are putative neurotransmitters (Baldessarini and Yorke, 1974).

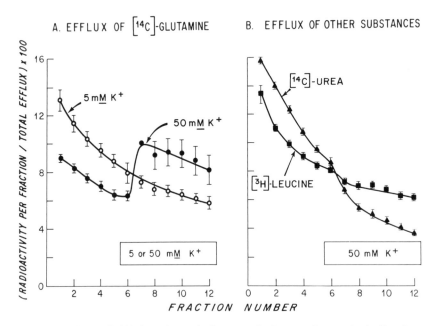

Figure 4.9 Release of [¹⁴C]-glutamine and other control substances from rat brain slices by 50 mM K⁺. Minces of rat forebrain were superfused in plastic chambers with a physiological medium followed by a medium in which Na⁺ was replaced by K⁺. The data are expressed as percentages of the total radioactivity released in each fraction. There was no release of radioactive urea or leucine.

Suggestions of the Models

If hepatic coma is due to the displacement of normal central transmitters or abnormal accumulations of metabolic products, then supplying greater amounts of the normal transmitters or their precursors might tend to restore a more normal functional status. Similarly, if abnormal amines or other products have accumulated in peripheral sympathetic nerve endings, restoration of normal transmitter stores should reverse the cardiovascular abnormalities associated with hepatic failure. Thus one would predict that an increase in peripheral vascular resistance should lead to a correction of any maldistribution of blood flow, a decreased demand for high cardiac output, and a subsequent alleviation of left-ventricular insufficiency and pulmonary congestion—all of which are common complications of severe liver failure.

The pharmacology of the adrenergic system places some constraints on the management of patients in hepatic failure. It is not useful merely to administer large doses of potent sympathomimetic amines. Such compounds enter the central nervous system very poorly and reach peripheral adrenergic terminals only with difficulty. Most of an administered dose of l-norepinephrine, for example, is rapidly metabolized, and that which does reach the appropriate neuroeffector junctions produces profound and poorly controllable α-adrenergic effects by direct postsynaptic action, with gangrene of the extremities a common complication of its prolonged intravenous administration. Nevertheless norepinephrine does have useful acute effects against the cardiovascular complications of hepatic failure. Interestingly, however, indirectly sympathomimetic amines (such as tyramine) are without effect, presumably because there is less norepinephrine available for release. Massive doses of metaraminol (a weak direct α-agonist) can also help to reverse the cardiovascular and renal dysfunctions in question, although the mental status is not altered (Fischer and Baldessarini, 1971; Fischer and James, 1972).

Alternatively the ability of L-dihydroxyphenylalanine (L-DOPA) to produce beneficial central neurological effects in patients with Parkinson's disease, and the treatment of hypertension with precursors (such as α-methyl-DOPA) of potential false transmitters, provide a basis for the suggestion that certain exogenous precursors can enter both peripheral adrenergic terminals and central catecholamine-containing nerve endings, where they can be converted to amine molecules. Therefore the administration of L-DOPA to patients in hepatic coma might result in the improvement of their central neurological status as well as their cardiovascular function. We have found that L-DOPA in moderately large doses can reverse the neuropsychiatric signs of hepatic coma in addition to improving the patient's circulatory status (Fischer and Baldessarini, 1971; Fischer and James, 1972). In contrast large doses of 5-hydroxytryptophan, the precursor of serotonin, do not have beneficial effects on the brain function of patients in precoma. Thus a treatment to facilitate the formation of serotonin in the brain and treatments that improved such patients' peripheral cardiovascular and renal status did not improve their neuropsychiatric status. When L-DOPA was added to their regimen, the coma of such patients often diminished within several hours. These clinical results are consistent with the hypothesis that adrenergic transmission may be abnormal in patients in hepatic failure and that these abnormalities may occur in the central nervous system as well as the periphery. We suggest that adrenergic transmission in the brain may be abnormal because of the accumulation of a variety of relatively impotent aromatic amines or amino acids at central nerve terminals.

Another aspect of animal models of hepatic encephalopathy is that they can be used to evaluate interventions known or suspected to be therapeutically useful in relation to the false-transmitter theory. For example, when L-DOPA was given to rats with portacaval anastomoses, the increased levels of serotonin present in their brains underwent a dramatic decrease, with a corresponding increase in the deaminated metabolite 5-hydroxyindoleacetic acid (Table 4.5). These results are consistent with the hypothesis that L-DOPA is converted to dopamine, which "flushes" serotonin from its storage sites and makes it more available to the action of MAO. In addition L-DOPA may have other effects, including interference with the synthesis of serotonin, and this action may become relatively more important over a longer time span, following the rapid displacing action which may occur acutely. We have observed a similar ability of L-DOPA to decrease the retention of labeled α-methyl-tyramine and its β-hydroxylated metabolite in the brain of the intact rat. This labeled compound may, in a sense, serve as a "model" for other peculiar amines; it is a poor substrate for MAO, it can pass the blood-brain barrier, and it can be studied in animals which are not treated with drugs or otherwise made abnormal by surgical interruption of the hepatic blood supply.

One other use of an animal model to test the effects of a treatment known to be helpful in the management of hepatic encephalopathy has been to treat rats with portacaval anastomoses with a poorly absorbed antibiotic in order to "sterilize" the gut (Table 4.6). In this case endogenous octopamine in the brain increased markedly (see Table 4.3), but when kanamycin was given by mouth, the level of this amine in the brain decreased sharply (Fischer et al., 1972). The antibiotic treatment had little effect on the normally low concentrations of octopamine in the brains of control rats exposed only to a "sham" surgical procedure.

While the correlation between a fall in the brain level of octopamine in

Table 4.6
Effects of intestinal sterilization on brain octopamine (ng/g $\pm$ S.E.M.)

	Octopamine
Sham operation (control)	7.3 $\pm$ 0.8
Sham + Kanamycin administered	6.9 $\pm$ 0.7
Portacaval shunt	28.7 $\pm$ 3.2*
Shunt + Kanamycin administered	15.2 $\pm$ 3.1

* $p < 0.01$ by t-test; $N \geq 6$.

the experimental model and the effectiveness of intestinal sterilization in the clinical situation is interesting, the interpretation of this finding is not simple. It is not clear how gut flora might influence the metabolism of amines in the brain. One possibility is that simple amines, for example phenethylamine, with limited polarity might be produced by the bacteria and made available to the portal circulation. Normally such products of the very active bacterial decarboxylases would be rapidly oxidized and inactivated by the liver parenchyma, but in the case of liver disease and with the associated shunting of portal blood directly into the systemic circulation (as well as in the animal surgical model), such amines would be available to the brain for local hydroxylation. Although it is possible that the brain can convert phenethylamine to tyramine, and it can β-hydroxylate tyramine to octopamine, it might be that tyramine produced in the gut reaches the brain if the normal blood-brain barrier to this phenolic amine is diminished as a consequence of the abnormal metabolic status of an animal with venous anastomoses.

Extensions and Summary
Whether the hypothesis we have presented is of relevance to other neurological or psychiatric illnesses is unclear. In addition to the asterixis and coma that commonly accompany severe hepatic failure, a variety of psychotic syndromes have also been described in such patients (Read et al., 1967), and the accumulation of false transmitters may be important in their pathophysiology. Possible connections between hepatic dysfunction and catatonia have also been suggested in the past (de Jong, 1945), and the ability of phenylethylamines to induce bizarre stereotyped behavior has been compared to certain phenomena seen in catatonia (Randrup and Munkvad, 1970). A disease which does have a marked

excess of circulating aromatic amino acids and an overproduction of phenylethylamines is phenylketonuria (Oates et al., 1963). Whether the neuropsychiatric aspects of this or any other disease due to heritable metabolic error may be partially related to the accumulation of false transmitters is still unknown. Since there are now many known metabolic errors and many putative neurotransmitters, the possibilities for future research along this line are quite broad.

Other examples of an excessive availability of aromatic amino acids or simple amines include the treatment of parkinsonism with L-DOPA and the use of amphetamines, both of which may result in profound behavioral changes, including psychotic reactions, in patients. Since L-DOPA can apparently lead to the excessive accumulation of dopamine in nondopaminergic neurons and since L-DOPA and the amphetamines can be converted to phenolic amine products that accumulate in the CNS in some species, it is possible that they may produce certain effects in the brain by a false-transmitter mechanism. For example, the well-known phenomenon of "tolerance" to the effects of the amphetamines might be due to the accumulation of their hydroxylated metabolites in central catecholaminergic nerve terminals, where they might be stored and released but have weak postsynaptic effects and thus act as false transmitters.

Examples of increased accumulations of probable false transmitters caused by decreased destruction of amines are perhaps most clearly provided by the chronic effects of MAO inhibitors (Kopin, 1968), although whether their antidepressant and psychotogenic effects may be partly mediated by increased accumulations of amines other than the catecholamines or serotonin in the CNS is not known. One intriguing possibility is that the reported decrease in activity of MAO in the blood platelets (a model of nerve endings?) of certain patients with severe idiopathic psychiatric illnesses might provide an opportunity for false-transmitter amines to accumulate and thereby to compromise the function of central aminergic synapses, if such enzyme deficiencies are in fact physiologically significant and if they occur in brain as well as in blood (Murphy, 1972; Wyatt et al., 1973). A summary of possible circumstances in which false transmitters might accumulate is shown in Table 4.7.

Table 4.7
Conditions under which false neurochemical transmitters might accumulate at nerve endings

A. *Increased precursor availability*	
1. Amino-acid therapy: L-DOPA, α-methyl-DOPA, α-methyl-*m*-tyrosine	
2. Amine therapy: amphetamines, tyramine, metaraminol	
3. Portacaval venous anastomosis: surgical or in liver disease	
4. Decreased hepatic utilization of amino acids due to toxins, drugs, or liver disease	
5. Metabolic error (e.g., phenylketonuria)	
B. *Decreased catabolism of amines*	
1. MAO inactivity: drug-induced or spontaneous	
2. Liver failure	

Our studies thus suggest that certain cardiovascular and renal complications of hepatic failure may be mediated by the dysfunction of the peripheral sympathetic nervous system. We propose that one mechanism for the dysfunction may be the accumulation of a variety of relatively inactive aromatic amines at nerve endings, caused by the increased availability of their precursors and the decreased catabolism of amines during hepatic failure. A similar mechanism in the CNS may underlie the neuropsychiatric complications of hepatic failure. The peripheral problems can be reversed by adrenergic compounds, and L-DOPA can reverse both peripheral and central dysfunctions. We suggest that the accumulation of false transmitters might also mediate a variety of other neuropsychiatric phenomena seen in states of inborn metabolic error or after the administration of certain drugs. An approach to the study of the relationships between neuropsychiatric disorders and neurotransmitter metabolism might therefore include a search for accumulations of nonfunctional structural analogues of any physiological transmitter in the nervous system.

It should be noted, finally, that the study of hepatic encephalopathy has been greatly assisted by the availability of animal models of clinical hepatic failure prepared by surgical shunting of the portal blood into the systemic circulation. Furthermore tissue slices and subcellular fractions rich in isolated nerve endings have also facilitated the laboratory study of the metabolism of amines and amino acids at the region of the synapse—an important region virtually inaccessible in the intact living brain.

References

Baldessarini, R. J. 1972. Biogenic amines and behavior. *Annu. Rev. Med.* 23:694–701.

Baldessarini, R. J. 1975. Amine metabolism in relation to affective disorders. In F. F. Flach and S. Draghi, eds., *The nature and treatment of depression.* New York: Wiley (in press).

Baldessarini, R. J., and Fischer, J. E. 1973. Serotonin metabolism in rat brain after surgical diversion of the portal venous circulation. *Nature [New Biol.]* 245:25–27.

Baldessarini, R. J., and Karobath, M. 1973. Biochemical physiology of central synapses. *Annu. Rev. Physiol.* 35:273–304.

Baldessarini, R. J., and Vogt, M. 1972. The regional release of aromatic amines from the brain of the rat *in vitro. J. Neurochem.* 19:755–761.

Baldessarini, R. J., and Yorke, C. 1974. Uptake and release of possible false transmitter amino acids by rat brain tissue. *J. Neurochem.* 23:839–848.

de Jong, H. H. 1945. *Experimental catatonia.* Baltimore: Williams & Wilkins.

Fischer, J. E. 1975. Acute hepatic failure, hepatic coma and the hepatorenal syndromes. In F. F. Becker, ed., *The molecular biology of liver disease.* New York: Decker (in press).

Fischer, J. E., and Baldessarini, R. J. 1971. False neurotransmitters and hepatic failure. *Lancet* ii:75–80.

Fischer, J. E., Horst, W. D., and Kopin, I. J. 1965. β-Hydroxylated sympathomimetic amines as false transmitters. *Br. J. Pharmacol.* 24:477–484.

Fischer, J. E., and James, J. H. 1972. Treatment of hepatic coma and hepatorenal syndrome. *Am. J. Surg.* 123:222–230.

Fischer, J. E., James, J. H., and Baldessarini, R. J. 1972. Changes in brain amines following portal flow diversion and acute hepatic coma: Effects of levodopa (L-DOPA) and intestinal sterilization. *Surg. Forum* 23:348–350.

Kety, S. S., and Matthysse, S., eds. 1972. *Prospects for research on schizophrenia. (Neurosci. Res. Program Bull.,* vol. 10, no. 4.)

Kopin, I. J. 1968. False adrenergic transmitters. *Annu. Rev. Pharmacol.* 8:377–394.

Murphy, D. L. 1972. Amine precursors, amines and false neurotransmitters in depressed patients. *Am. J. Psychiatry* 129:141–148.

Oates, J. A., Nirenberg, P. Z., Jepson, J. B., Sjoerdsma, A., and Udenfriend, S. 1963. Conversion of phenylalanine to phenethylamine in patients with phenylketonuria. *Proc. Soc. Exp. Biol. Med.* 112:1078–1081.

Phyllis, J. W. 1970. *The pharmacology of synapses.* Oxford: Pergamon.

Randrup, A., and Munkvad, I. 1970. Biochemical, anatomical and psychological investigations of stereotyped behavior induced by amphetamines. In E. Costa and S. Garattini, eds., *Amphetamines and related compounds.* New York: Raven.

Read, A. E., Sherlock, S., Laidlaw, J., and Walker, J. G. 1967. The neuropsychiatric syndromes associated with chronic liver disease and an extensive portal-systemic collateral circulation. *Q. J. Med.* 36:135–150.

Warren, K. S., and Schenker, S. 1964. Effect of an inhibitor of glutamine synthesis (methionine sulfoximine) on ammonia toxicity and metabolism. *J. Lab. Clin. Med.* 64:442–449.

Wyatt, R. J., Murphy, D. L., Belmaker, R., Donnelly, C., Cohen, S., and Pollin, W. 1973. Reduced monoamine oxidase activity in platelets: A possible genetic marker for vulnerability to schizophrenia. *Science* 179:916–918.

5

Tissue- and Cell-Culture Models in the Study of Neurotransmitter and Synaptic Function

Harvey M. Shein

A large body of basic and neuropharmacological research suggests that alterations in neurotransmitter (catecholamine and indoleamine) metabolism at brain synapses are of importance in the pathophysiology of affective as well as schizophrenic disorders (Schildkraut and Kety, 1967; Matthysse and Kety, 1972). Sufficient evidence has accumulated to define these concepts and to support their heuristic usefulness as working hypotheses, so that it has now become both feasible and essential to explore their implications at the cellular, molecular, and genetic levels. Although the neurotransmitter-dysfunction hypotheses now seem to be most promising, it still remains quite possible that alternative or additional kinds of brain dysfunction, such as aberrations in specific brain cell structures or in the genetic control of neuronal development, structure, or function, will eventually be found to be etiologically involved in the pathophysiology of the psychoses.

A major lesson of neurobiological research in the last decade has been that important problems are most effectively formulated, defined, and solved through a close collaboration among pharmacologists, physiologists, anatomists, and geneticists. Accordingly it is necessary to approach the study of the basic biology of the psychoses with simplified experimental systems that can model, not only neurotransmitter functions, but also developmental, structural, and genetic aspects of neuronal and glial functions. It is for these reasons that techniques of cell and tissue culture, which provide in vitro experimental systems of less complexity than the intact nervous system for the analysis of neurotransmitter-related and other neurobiological problems at basic biological and biochemical levels, offer unique opportunities for studies of the basic pathophysiological mechanisms of the psychoses.

This work was supported in part by U.S. Public Health Service Research Grant NS 06610.

Techniques of cell and tissue culture can be said to provide "models" for the study of normal and disordered central-nervous-system neurotransmitter and synaptic functions in the sense that these less complex experimental systems can be used to represent such functions at both the tissue level (by organ cultures of nervous and neuroendocrine tissues) and the cellular level (by dispersed cultures of "pure" and mixed brain cell types).

Tissues and cells can be cultured in vitro in a variety of ways: by organ culture, in which tissue fragments or entire organs are explanted and maintained in vitro; by dispersed cell culture, in which cells are first separated by gentle enzymatic treatment of the tissues and the dispersed cells are then maintained or propagated in vitro; and by reaggregation culture, in which dispersed cells from one or more immature tissues are maintained in vitro under conditions of rotary shaking such that the cells reaggregate and develop into "tissues" in vitro. Both normal and neoplastic nervous and nonnervous tissues and cells can be cultured in vitro by such techniques. In addition single normal or neoplastic cells growing in dispersed cell cultures can be isolated and propagated as genetically homogeneous cell populations, called *cloned cell lines.*

This chapter discusses the present uses and the potential usefulness of tissue- and cell-culture models for the study of central neurotransmitter and synaptic functions in the context of illustrative model systems. Some of the significant questions important to neuropsychiatry that can be addressed by these models are—

1. the physiological and genetic control mechanisms of neurotransmitter function and receptor response in neurons and glia;
2. the definition of the characteristics of neuronal and glial cell types maintained in pure cultures;
3. the effects of various neurotransmitters and pharmacological agents on the plasticity and physiology of identifiable neurons at synaptic junctions;
4. the physiological and genetic control mechanisms of neuronal and glial development and interaction (e.g., cell proliferation, migration, the formation of specific functional connections).

Each of the model systems now available or under development is more useful for study of some of these questions than for others. Thus the most useful applications of tissue and cell cultures typically employ a variety of models, each used to analyze those aspects of the problem under study for which that model is best suited. Because of this mutually complementary use of tissue- and cell-culture models, the presentation that follows begins with a description of problems that can now be studied in relatively well-defined systems and then proceeds to describe technical developments of these models and additional models now under development that would permit other significant problems to be studied. Tables 5.2 and 5.3 below summarize the important questions that can now be addressed in one or another model system and illustrate the necessity for appropriate complementary use of different tissue- or cell-culture systems in exploring these questions. The reader should continuously refer to these two tables to maintain a sense of continuity in regard to the important problems that are accessible to exploration by each of the tissue- and cell-culture systems that will be described.

Available Tissue- and Cell-Culture Systems

Organ Cultures of Pineal Gland and Sympathetic Ganglia   Organ cultures of rat pineal gland and of rat or chick sympathetic ganglia have been used to model complementary aspects of adrenergic-neuron functions. The pineal gland models aspects of adrenergic input that induce hormonal synthesis and release, and the ganglia model aspects of adrenergic output (synthesis, storage, and release) in response to cholinergic input.

The rat pineal gland in situ synthesizes serotonin and melatonin from tryptophan in complementary diurnal rhythms (Wurtman, Axelrod, and Kelly, 1968) and is innervated exclusively by adrenergic neurons that synapse directly on the pineal parenchymal cells (Figure 5.1). It has been shown by use of pineal organ cultures, and later confirmed by in vivo studies, that norepinephrine activates β-adrenergic receptors on pinealocytes and thereby stimulates adenylate cyclase and increases intracellular cyclic adenosine monophosphate (cAMP) content. The increased intracellular cAMP in turn induces an enormously increased synthesis of the enzyme that N-acetylates pineal serotonin (N-acetyltransferase, NAT), thereby greatly increasing melatonin synthesis and decreasing serotonin synthesis (Shein, 1971). Rat pineal organ cultures thus provide a model that is isomorphic to the in situ pineal in respect to the transsynaptic mechanisms by which norepinephrine controls pineal serotonin and melatonin synthesis (Table 5.1).

Accordingly these cultures provide an ideal model system for analysis of the molecular mechanisms by which catecholamines interact with β-adrenergic receptors and the cAMP system in postsynaptic cells to induce synthesis of a specific new enzyme. This model system has, for example, recently been used (Deguchi and Axelrod, 1974) to show that denervation superinduction of NAT by norepinephrine requires continuous norepinephrine stimulation of the β-adrenergic receptor on

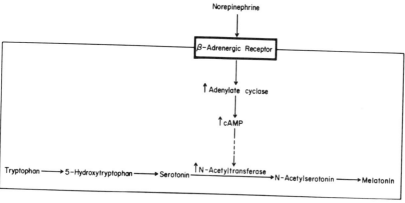

Figure 5.1 Control of melatonin synthesis by norepinephrine in rat pineal organ culture.

Table 5.1
Adrenegic postsynaptic actions on rat pineal indole metabolism modeled in organ cultures

1. Effects of norepinephrine (NE) on indole metabolism

    a. ↑ Adenylate cyclase activity
    b. ↑↑Intracellular cAMP synthesis
    c. ↑↑Synthesis of serotonin N-acetyltransferase
    d. ↑↑Synthesis of melatonin
    e. ↓↓Synthesis of serotonin

2. Effects of adrenergic blocking and mimicking agents on indole metabolism

    a. All effects of NE (1a-1e) are prevented by β but not by α adrenergic receptor blocking agents
    b. All effects of NE (1a-1e) are mimicked by the specific β-receptor stimulator isoproterenol
    c. Only intracellular effects of NE (1c-1e) are mimicked by dibutyryl cAMP or theophylline

the pineal cell, and must be due to changes between the receptor and the action site of cAMP inasmuch as the superinduction is not mimicked by added cAMP. These investigators have further shown that the induction of denervation supersensitivity in the pineal β-adrenergic receptor must be due to the absence of neurotransmitter caused by denervation inasmuch as repeated injection of isoproterenol to denervated rats prevents superinduction of NAT in vivo, and repeated injection of isoproterenol to intact rats results in a much lower increase in NAT activity in cultured pineals in response to added isoproterenol.

In contrast to the pineal gland, sympathetic ganglia are innervated in situ by cholinergic neurons. These ganglia can be excised and maintained in organ culture for weeks or months, during which time the adrenergic neurons develop extensive axonal processes if nerve growth factor is added to the nutrient medium. These axonal processes contain microtubules and large granular vesicles and develop "functional" synapses when permitted to grow into contact with tissues (such as the smooth muscle cells of the iris) that are sympathetically innervated in vivo. These axonal sprouts also exhibit mechanisms of active uptake of norepinephrine, release of norepinephrine in response to electrical depolarization, and blockage or enhancement of norepinephrine release in response to drugs, that appear to be identical to those observed in situ. Kopin and coworkers (1974) have investigated induction of catecholamine (CA)-synthesizing enzymes in organ-cultured sympathetic ganglia (Figure 5.2). They have found that depolarization by high levels

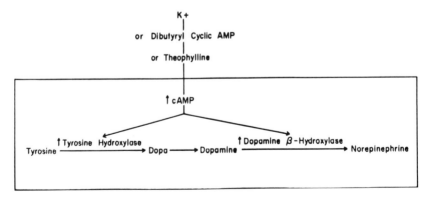

Figure 5.2 Control of catecholamine synthesis in sympathetic-ganglion culture and adrenergic-neuroblastoma cell culture.

of potassium, or addition of dibutyryl cAMP or theophylline, produces increased activity of both tyrosine hydroxylase (TH) and dopamine β-hydroxylase (DBH) that is blocked by inhibition of protein synthesis. These results suggest but do not yet prove that cAMP may be involved in the induction of these enzymes and possibly also in the transneuronal induction of these enzymes that is observed in vivo. Organ cultures of sympathetic ganglia thus provide a model that appears to be isomorphic to the in situ ganglia in respect to axonal-process formation, synapse formation, norepinephrine uptake, storage, and release, and control of CA-synthesizing enzymes. Accordingly the sympathetic-ganglion cultures appear to provide a particularly powerful model system for analysis of the molecular mechanisms underlying both short- and long-term control of these phenomena in adrenergic neurons.

Cloned Neuroblastoma and Glioma Cell Cultures   Dispersed cultures of cloned neuroblastoma and glioma cell lines that retain certain differentiated functions of normal neurons and glial cells have been used to study a wide range of biochemical, physiological, and developmental characteristics of these nervous cell types and to analyze genetic control mechanisms for these characteristics (Rosenberg, 1972). In addition to nervous cell type specificity and relative genetic homogeneity, these cloned cell lines offer the advantages that the cells can be grown in as large quantities as are desired and that mutant clones with altered differentiated functions can be selected by appropriate conditions of culture. The fact that these cell lines are neoplastic and are grown separately from other nervous-tissue cell types has necessitated great caution in extrapolation to normal cell function and structure in situ. However, the use of cultures of pure nervous cell types, even if neoplastic, has provided for the first time experimental systems in which there is at least the opportunity to delineate specific neuronal or glial cell functions that are independent of the presence of other nervous cell types. In spite of the problems and limitations much significant new information has already been obtained from studies employing these systems.

Studies with dispersed neuroblastoma cells have utilized cloned cell lines derived from the Bar Harbor C-1300 mouse neuroblastoma that exhibit neuron-like differentiation when cultivated in vitro (Tables 5.2

Table 5.2
Neuronal neurotransmitter (NT)-related functions in organ and cell-culture systems

	Type of Organ or Cell Culture System					
1. Cell receptor response to specific NT's	Symp. gang. o.c.	Symp. gang. d.c.	Brain or spinal cord d.c.	Neuro-blastoma d.c.	Invert. gang. o.c.	Invert. neuron. d.c.
a. Action potential	+	+	+	+	+	+
b. Induction of cAMP synthesis	+	+	+	+	?	?
c. Induction of specific NT enzyme(s) synthesis	+	+	+	+	?	?
2. Uptake, storage and release of NT's						
a. Active uptake	+	+?	?	O	?	?
b. Storage in intracellular granules	+	+?	?	±?	?	?
c. Release in response to electrical depolarization or drugs	+	?	?	O?	?	?
3. Synthesis of NT-related enzymes						
a. All enzymes in pathway remain active in culture	+	+	?	+?	+?	?
b. Mutants available in which only certain enzymes remain active	O	O	?	+	?	?
c. Induction by drugs that ↑intracellular cAMP	+	?	?	+	?	?

o.c. = organ culture
d.c. = dispersed cell culture

Table 5.3
Neuronal survival, axon formation, axon maturity, and capacity for normal histogenesis in organ and cell-culture systems

	Type of Organ or Cell Culture System						
1. Neuronal survival in culture requires added:	Brain rotation culture	Neuro-blastoma d.c.	Symp. gang. o.c.	Symp. gang. d.c.	Brain spinal cord d.c.	Invert. gang. o.c.	Invert. neuron d.c.
a. Nerve growth factor	O	O	O	+	O	O	O
b. "Glial" or other non-neuronal cell factors	+	O	O	+	+	O	+
2. Axon formation in response to:							
a. Nerve growth factor	?	±	+	+	?	O	O
b. Drugs that ↑intracellular cAMP levels	?	+	?	?	+?	O	O
c. BUDR, X-irradiation, or serum-free-medium	?	+	?	?	?	O	O
d. "Glial" or other non-neuronal cell factors	?	+	?	?	+?	+	+
3. Axon Maturity: Capacity for synapse formation							
a. Synapse formation by EM criteria	+	O	+	?	+	+	+
b. Synapse formation by neurophysio. criteria	?	O	+	+	+	+	+
4. Histogenetic and biochemical development							
a. Normal neuronal migration and alignment	+	O	NA	O	O	NA	O
b. Formation of approximately normal histogenetic tissue	+	O	NA	O	O	NA	O
c. Capacity to develop de novo or further mature without specific additives:							
(1) Myelin formation	+	O	NA	?	?	NA	O
(2) Synapse formation	+	O	+	?	+	+	±
(3) Specific activity of NT-related enzymes	+	O	O	O	+	O	O
(4) Synthesis of cAMP in response to added NT	+	O	O	O	O	O	O

o.c. = organ culture
d.c. = dispersed cell culture

and 5.3). Certain of these mouse neuroblastoma clones extend long axonal processes containing neurofilaments, neurotubules, and large, granular, dense-core vesicles when cultivated in a serum-free medium in the presence of a factor released into the medium of cultured cloned glioma cells, or in the presence of dibutyryl cAMP, 5-bromodeoxyuridine, or X-irradiation (Table 5.3). Clones have also been selected that do not put out axons under any of these stimuli. The molecular mechanisms responsible for inducing the morphological differentiation remain undefined but appear to be different for each of the effective agents listed. A large portion of the neuroblastoma cells from most clones that extend long axons exhibit action potentials after electrical stimulation or application of acetylcholine, and these action potentials exhibit neuron-like sensitivity to blocking agents. Most of the clones contain enzymes that inactivate acetylcholine (i.e., acetylcholinesterase) and catecholamines (i.e., catechol-O-methyltransferase, COMT). The specific activity of both of these enzymes is much higher in nondividing cells. Clones have been selected that are exclusively "adrenergic" in that they have high activities of tyrosine hydroxylase (TH) in the absence of choline acetyltransferase (CAT) activity, or exclusively "cholinergic" in that they have high CAT activity in the absence of TH activity. Clones have also been found in which the cells are both "adrenergic" and "cholinergic" in that they have high levels of both TH and CAT, or in which the cells have electrically excitable axons but lack both TH and CAT. Dibutyryl cAMP, which inhibits cell division and induces morphological differentiation in mouse neuroblastoma cells, also increases TH and acetylcholinesterase activity in these cells. In adrenergic clones that contain dopamine β-hydroxylase (DBH), addition of dibutyryl cAMP has been reported to stimulate DBH activity during the period of cell division. It is worth noting that these observations of dibutyryl-cAMP-induced increase in TH and DBH activity in cloned neuroblastoma cells agree with findings in sympathetic-ganglion cultures (Figure 5.2).

   Nirenberg and associates have attempted to explore the mechanisms controlling gene expression of neuron-specific functions in neuroblastoma cells by studies using somatic cell hybrids (Minna, Glazer, and Nirenberg, 1972). By fusing mouse neuroblastoma cells with those of a mouse fibroblast cell line (L cells) to form cell lines containing both parental genomes, these investigators have shown that certain neuronal properties, including the formation of neurites, the presence of electrically excitable membranes, and the synthesis of acetyl-cholinesterase, can be expressed in neuroblastoma/L-cell hybrid cells and that hybrid clones with specific defects in neuronal function can also be readily obtained. Specific karyological analysis to permit localization of the structural genes for the neuronal properties expressed in the hybrids to specific mouse chromosomes was not possible in these studies because all of the cell lines employed for the fusion studies were mouse cells. However, it can be anticipated that future studies of this type employing hybrid cells derived from human neuroblastoma cells and mouse fibroblast cells will permit localization of the structural genes for the differentiated neuronal characteristics expressed in the hybrids to specific human chromosomes. The nuclei of human/mouse hybrid cells gradually lose the human chromosomes upon subcultivation, so that serial karyological analyses done in parallel with analyses of any neuron-specific function expressed in human-neuroblastoma/mouse-fibroblast hybrid cells can enable one to determine which human chromosome(s) is (are) associated with the loss of the capacity of the hybrid cells to perform the function of interest.

Dispersed cell cultures of cloned rat and human glioma cell lines that synthesize the nervous-system-specific S-100 protein have been used to clarify biochemical and pharmacological aspects of glial cell function (Rosenberg, 1972). Some of these cloned glioma lines contain 2′, 3′ cAMP-3 phosphohydrolase, an enzyme thought previously to be a marker for myelin. Other enzymes present in these cloned cells include COMT and monoamine oxidase (MAO). Addition of cortisol or epinephrine to these cells has been found to induce synthesis of the enzyme glycerol phosphate dehydrogenase.

More importantly, addition of norepinephrine or isoproterenol to cultured cloned glioma cells has been shown to induce, via interaction with β-adrenergic receptors, a remarkably rapid, large, and sustained increase in the intracellular levels of cAMP (Figure 5.3). Addition of norepinephrine to one such cloned glial line has also been found to induce synthesis of a specific molecular form of the enzyme, cAMP phosphodiesterase, that metabolizes cAMP (Uzunov, Shein, and Weiss, 1973). The induction of cAMP in glial cells by addition of a neurotransmitter has prompted the hypothesis that neurons may "communicate" with glial cells using this mechanism. This possibility has recently been supported by the finding that the addition of norepinephrine to a medium of cloned rat glioma cell cultures produces a marked increase in glycogenolysis in these cells that is thought to be mediated by increased intracellular cAMP (Figure 5.3).

Tissue- and Cell-Culture Models Now under Development

Dispersed Cell Cultures from Ganglia, Spinal Cord, and Brain   As was previously noted, cloned neuroblastoma cells in culture exhibit many characteristics of normal sympathetic and cholinergic neurons. However, these neoplastic cells have not been shown as yet to exhibit certain particularly important neuronal characteristics such as synapse formation, specific active cellular uptake of neurotransmitters, and binding and release of transmitters from intracellular storage sites (Table 5.2). Accordingly intense investigatory effort is now being directed toward developing techniques for dispersed cell cultivation of normal neurons and glia derived from sympathetic ganglia, dorsal-root ganglia,

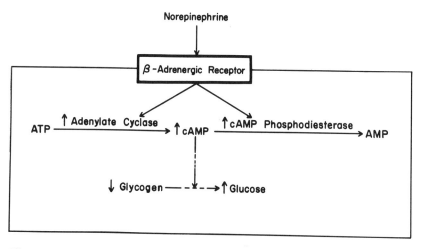

Figure 5.3 Effects of norepinephrine on cAMP and glycogen metabolism in cloned astrocytoma cells.

and spinal-cord and brain tissues of embryonic chicks and mice (Fischbach, Fambraugh, and Nelson, 1973).

By use of gentle trypsinization or mechanical dissociation, dispersed cell cultures containing reproducible mixtures of viable neurons and glia can now be obtained from each of these tissues and maintained for several weeks in vitro. Neurons in these cultures form dense, spontaneously active synaptic networks in which both excitatory and inhibitory synapses have been identified over cell bodies and dendrites and in which long sequences of evoked potentials have been recorded by stimulation of identified cells and processes. Synaptic boutons are readily located in these cultures by electron microscopy and in the living cells by light microscopy. Not only do neurons in such cultures form synapses with other neurons, they also form physiologically active synapses with dissociated muscle cells added to the cultures. It has been further shown that some degree of specificity of neuronal synapse formation is retained in these cultures (sensory neurons, for example, will not form synapses with added muscle cells).

It is apparent that, even in their present relatively primitive stage of development, these dispersed cell cultures from ganglia, spinal cord, and brain provide uniquely useful in vitro systems for study of the effects of various neurotransmitters, blocking agents, and electrical and chemical stimuli on the plasticity and physiology of individually identifiable axon boutons at synaptic junctions. However, the characterization of the differentiated functions of neurons in these cultures as isomorphic to differentiated functions of corresponding neurons in vivo remains incomplete. The retention of certain important neuronal functions has not yet been demonstrated in these cultures, and the role of specific neurotransmitters in mediating the observed transsynaptic evoked potentials has not as yet been defined in most of these culture systems. For example, studies have not as yet been reported that establish whether neurons in these dispersed cell cultures retain specialized uptake, storage, and release mechanisms for specific neurotransmitters (Table 5.2). It has been shown for dispersed mouse brain cell cultures that there is a progressive increase over time in the activity of choline acetyltransferase and glutamate decarboxylase, two putative neuron-specific "marker" enzymes for the neurotransmitters acetylcholine and GABA (Table 5.2). However, except in studies with mixed cultures of spinal-cord and muscle cells, in which acetylcholine has clearly been shown to be the active neurotransmitter, it has not been demonstrated with cultures from brain or spinal cord that increased amounts of these enzymes represent further biochemical differentiation in these neurons in vitro or that either acetylcholine or GABA functions as a physiologically active neurotransmitter in these cultures.

All of the dispersed cell cultures of vertebrate nervous tissues just discussed and presently available include nonneuronal cells in addition to neurons. For many types of investigation of the molecular mechanisms of normal neuronal development, structure, and function at the cellular level, pure cell cultures of "normal" neurons of a given neurotransmitter-producing type would be more useful as experimental systems. In regard to the technical problems and prospects for developing such systems, it is of importance that recent observations indicate a neuronal requirement for nonneuronal cell products (Table 5.3). For example, most neurons dissociated from sympathetic or dorsal-root ganglia do not survive in culture, even in the presence of nerve growth factor (NGF), unless adequate numbers of glial cells are also present in the culture. Recently it has been shown that additional glial cells can substitute for NGF in enhancing the survival and morphological differentiation of neurons in dissociated spinal-ganglia cultures (Burnham, Raiborn, and Varon, 1972). It has also been reported that addition of an undefined factor released into the culture medium by cloned glioma cells stimulates morphological differentiation of cloned neuroblastoma cells in culture (Monard et al., 1973). Taken together these observations suggest that normal neurons require one or more factors released by glial cells in order to survive and differentiate adequately in culture in the absence of nonneuronal cells. It appears, therefore, that the availability of pure cultures of differentiated normal neurons from vertebrates must await the further study of these presently unidentified supporting factors provided by glial cells.

The observations of Levi-Montalcini and Aloe (1972) on cultures of invertebrate neurons are also consistent with the concept of neuronal dependence on nonneuronal factors. These investigators have recently prepared cultures consisting exclusively of invertebrate neurons (from ganglia of the embryonic cockroach) by using a technique of mechanical dissociation that selectively destroys the noneuronal cells. However, in these cultures also, the presence of nonneuronal factors is apparently essential for continued biochemical and morphological differentiation of the cultured neurons (Table 5.3). Thus the dissociated glia-free neurons produce a dense axonal network, continue to synthesize neurotransmitter-related enzymes (choline acetyltransferase and acetylcholinesterase), and form synaptic connections only if the neurons are cultured in the presence of ganglion explants or in the presence of other tissues from the cockroach (Schlapfer, Haywood, and Barondes, 1972).

Reaggregating Cultures of Dissociated Brain Cells   An ideal combined cell- and tissue-culture model for study of the molecular mechanisms underlying neuronal differentiation, migration, and the formation of functionally appropriate synaptic connections in brain tissue, would start with dissociated, pure populations of developmentally immature neurons, glia, and other cell types comprising a given brain tissue (e.g., cerebellum) and would then provide techniques for reaggregation of the dissociated cells in vitro to form brain tissues, which would develop in a normal or abnormal manner depending on the cellular characteristics and relative proportions (numbers) of the starting cell types. As has been already noted, methods have not yet been developed for separating vertebrate neuronal cell types from nonneuronal brain cell types so that they remain viable in culture. Nevertheless studies in which techniques of tissue reaggregation by rotation culture have been applied to dissociated mixtures of brain cell types have already demonstrated that reaggregation-culture techniques provide important new experimental systems for the analysis of developmental and genetic aspects of neurotransmitter- and synapse-related problems (Garber, 1972).

For example, it has been shown that if dispersed cells from the hippocampus of the isocortex of embryonic (18 days' gestation) mouse brains are cultured in flasks in a rotary shaker, the various cell types form aggregates with a histogenetic pattern closely resembling normal hippocampi of isocortical architecture (Table 5.3). By contrast, when dispersed cells from the isocortex of developing brains from mutant "reeler" mice of the same gestational age are maintained in rotary culture for the same period, the cellular architecture of neurons in the aggregates is disorganized, much as it is in the isocortex of these mutant mice in situ, strongly suggesting that the mutant-mouse grain neurons have a genetically determined defect in an intrinsic cellular function that permits normal neurons to achieve normal migration and alignment during development. It has not as yet been investigated whether this genetic defect in reeler mutant neurons is associated with defects in the development of neurotransmitter-related functions in these neurons.

The applicability of presently available reaggregating brain cell cultures as a model system for such studies has been recently confirmed (Seeds and Vatter, 1971; Seeds and Gilman, 1971) by the following evidence for continued morphological and biochemical differentiation in reaggregating cell cultures from embryonic mouse brains (Table 5.3): (1) Upon electron microscopic examination, the brain-cell aggregates show the presence of synapses that mature and increase in number during culture. (2) Myelination of axons is observed to develop in the aggregates after several weeks in culture. (3) The specific activities of several neuron-associated enzymes (choline acetyltransferase, acetyl-cholinesterase, and glutamate decarboxylase) increase in the aggregates during culture. (4) Norepinephrine causes a marked (fourfold to sixfold) increase in intracellular cAMP levels in the brain aggregate after nine days in culture, similar to the response observed in four-day-postnatal rat brain slices, but dissimilar to the lack of response observed in embryonic rat brain slices.

Can Cell-Culture Techniques Be Directly Applied to the Study of Psychoses in Patients?
In a symposium devoted to biological models in psychiatric research it seems appropriate to conclude a discussion of the use of tissue- and cell-culture models for the study of neurotransmitter and synaptic functions by considering the question of whether cell-culture techniques can be applied directly to the clinical study of psychoses. We have already emphasized that a large body of evidence suggests that alterations of catecholamine (CA) function may be involved in the pathophysiology of the affective disorders and the schizophrenias.

However, in investigations in man of central CA-related processes at the cellular level, one cannot employ direct experimental manipulation of brain tissues, so that one must at present employ indirect analyses that make use of body fluids or blood-tissue components. Nevertheless, despite the severe experimental limitations of these indirect methods, recent studies of MAO in platelets from bipolar depressives, of COMT in erythrocytes from unipolar and bipolar depressives, and of MAO in platelets from schizophrenic patients, suggest that the altered activities of these enzymes in these peripheral tissue sources may represent genetic "markers" for vulnerability to these disorders (Dunner et al., 1971). It is not known whether these findings are incidentally related to the actual pathogenic mechanisms of the disorders or whether they represent generalized malfunctions that occur in most or all peripheral tissues, as well as in the brain tissues, of these patients and that may possibly be related to the primary disorders.

One way of clarifying these questions is to study the functions of these CA-related enzymes in additional peripheral tissues and, where possible, in brain tissues from "normal" controls and from patients with affective disorders and schizophrenia. Skin biopsy is a benign and simple procedure which yields, not only material for immediate enzyme assay, but also, via well-defined cell-culture techniques, essentially unlimited quantities of multiplying, apparently "normal," nonneoplastic human skin fibroblasts of stable karyotype which are suitable both for comparative biochemical and pharmacological studies and for genetic-linkage analyses (i.e., for karyological studies on hybrid cells formed by fusion of the human skin fibroblasts and rodent cells). Similarly, fresh, unfixed brain fragments obtained shortly after death from normals and from patients with schizophrenia and affective disorders who die by suicide or accidental causes can also be prepared by well-defined cell-culture techniques to yield, in addition to material for immediate enzyme assay, dispersed cell cultures of neuroglial cells that have the same potential as the skin cell cultures for comparative biochemical, pharmacological, and genetic-linkage studies.

It is appropriate to recall, in support of the application of cell cultures of skin and glia to the study of disorders in which the primary dysfunctions are most likely located primarily in central neurons, that many human neurological diseases have already been described in which the essential metabolic abnormality has been found to be present in skin tissue and in skin fibroblasts in cell culture, despite the fact that the destructive expression of these disease processes is solely or primarily restricted to brain tissue. Thus important neurological disorders in which the specific enzyme abnormality or deficiency has been identified through the use of skin-fibroblast cell cultures include the diseases of Tay-Sachs, Gaucher, and Niemann-Pick, and also metachromatic leukodystrophy (Brady, 1970).

The principal significance of such investigations is that they would make available for the first time somatic cell lines from persons documented (as well as can now be done) as "normal," bipolar depressive, and schizophrenic. They would thereby provide an invaluable experimental tool and resource for the study of biochemical and pharmacological aspects and genetic linkages of presently claimed and future putative "markers" for these disorders as they are identified.

Conclusion

This chapter has presented an interpretive survey of the present status and potentialities of tissue- and cell-culture models for basic studies of neurotransmitter and synaptic functions. It can be anticipated with confidence that, as further evidence accumulates to implicate disordered neurotransmitter and synaptic functions in the pathophysiology of the psychoses, basic investigations in this area will make progressively greater use of the unique experimental opportunities offered by tissue- and cell-culture models for the experimental analysis of pertinent pharmacological, ultrastructural, and genetic mechanisms at cellular and molecular levels.

References

Brady, R. O. 1970. Cerebral lipodoses. *Annu. Rev. Med.* 21:317–334.

Burnham, P., Raiborn, C., and Varon, S. 1972. Replacement of nerve-growth factor by ganglionic non-neuronal cells for the survival *in vitro* of dissociated ganglionic neurons. *Proc. Natl. Acad. Sci. U.S.A.* 69:3556–3560.

Deguchi, T., and Axelrod, J. 1974. Role of β-adrenergic receptor in the control of serotonin N-acetyltransferase in rat pineal. In E. Usdin and S. Snyder, eds., *Frontiers in catecholamine research: Third international catecholamine symposium.* New York: Pergamon.

Dunner, D. L., Cohen, C. K., Gershon, E. S., and Goodwin, F. K. 1971. Differential catechol-O-methyl transferase activity in unipolar and bipolar affective illness. *Arch. Gen. Psychiatry* 25:348–353.

Fischbach, G. D., Fambraugh, D., and Nelson, P. G. 1973. Discussion on neuron and muscle cell cultures. *Fed. Proc.* 1636–1642.

Garber, B. B. 1972. Brain histogenesis *in vitro*. Reconstruction of brain tissue from dissociated cells. *In Vitro* 8:167–174.

Kopin, I. J., Berv, K. R., and Webb, J. G. 1974. Organ culture of sympathetic ganglia. In E. Usdin and S. Snyder, eds., *Frontiers in catecholamine research: Third international catecholamine symposium.* New York: Pergamon.

Levi-Montalcini, R., and Aloe, L. 1972. Neuronal nets and nerve cell interactions in insect systems. *In Vitro* 8:178–191.

Matthysse, S., and Kety, S. S., eds. 1972. *Prospects for research in schizophrenia. (Neurosci. Res. Program Bull.,* vol. 10, no. 4.)

Minna, J., Glazer, D., and Nirenberg, M. 1972. Genetic dissection of neural properties using somatic cell hybrids. *Nature [New Biol.]* 235:225–231.

Monard, D., Solomon, F., Reutsch, M., and Gysin, R. 1973. Glia-induced morphological differentiation in neuroblastoma cells. *Proc. Natl. Acad. Sci. U.S.A.* 70:1894–1897.

Rosenberg, R. N. 1972. Neuronal and glial enzyme studies in cell culture. *In Vitro* 8:194–204.

Schildkraut, J. J., and Kety, S. S. 1967. Biogenic amines and emotion. *Science* 156:21–30.

Schlapfer, W. T., Haywood, P., and Barondes, S. H. 1972. Cholinesterase and choline acetyltransferase activities develop in whole explant but not in dissociated cell cultures of cockroach brain. *Brain Res.* 39:540–544.

Seeds, N. W., and Gilman, A. G. 1971. Norepinephrine stimulated increase of cyclic AMP levels in developing mouse brain cell cultures. *Science* 174:292.

Seeds, N. W., and Vatter, A. E. 1971. Synaptogenesis in reaggregating brain cell culture. *Proc. Natl. Acad. Sci. U.S.A.* 68:3219–3272.

Shein, H. M. 1971. Control of melatonin synthesis by noradrenaline in rat pineal organ cultures. In G. E. W. Wolstenholme and J. Knight, eds., *The pineal gland.* London: Churchill, Livingstone.

Uzunov, P., Shein, H. M., and Weiss, B. 1973. Cyclic AMP phosphodiesterase in cloned astrocytoma cells: Norepinephrine induces a specific enzyme form. *Science* 180:304–306.

Wurtman, R. J., Axelrod, J., and Kelly, D. E. 1968. *The pineal.* New York: Academic Press.

6

Central Dopaminergic Neurons: A Model for Predicting the Efficacy of Putative Antipsychotic Drugs?

Benjamin S. Bunney and George K. Aghajanian

"When I was seven something strange happened to me. I became afraid to leave home for fear I would die if my mother was out of my sight. I realized that I was different from other people. When company would come over I'd pretend I had to study and lock myself in my room. Sometimes I'd hide in the closet or under the bed . . . I never had friends; I was always afraid of being hurt somehow, I guess I had lots of imaginary friends, though. My best friend was the P.D. (Prime Deceiver) who was responsible for controlling all that happened to me. I saw people as automatons on a conveyor belt forever passing in review before the P.D. I saw myself as a mutant form of one of these automatons. You I thought of as D.B.M. (Dr. Bunney Machine). You were a machine with a cord running from your back to an electrical outlet behind you. I could control you by unplugging you whenever I wanted to. I could never look at you because when I did your face became distorted, mutilated, with blood all over it.

"People often became unreal, like shadows. I felt unreal too. I used to wear a goat bell around my neck tucked inside my clothes which would ring when I walked and reminded me I was alive. Before I got the bell I used to walk around in the wintertime without gloves so I could feel the pain from the cold, and often I would hold my hand over an open flame just to feel something and to know that I existed."

The above are a few of the thoughts and actions related (to B.S.B.) by a 25-year-old female schizophrenic after four months of treatment with an antipsychotic medication.

When this patient first appeared for treatment she was frightened, anxious, unable to function either at work or at home, and, of course, extremely unhappy. She was bizarre in both appearance and mannerism, and her thoughts were difficult to follow because of blocking, looseness of association, and flight of ideas. For a while the patient refused

B. S. Bunney and G. K. Aghajanian, Departments of Psychiatry and Pharmacology, Yale University School of Medicine and the Connecticut Mental Health Center, New Haven, CT.

medication, and her clinical status became worse. However, she finally agreed to take the antipsychotic drug thioridazine (mellaril). Within two weeks she was able to communicate quite clearly and her bizarre thoughts and mannerisms had diminished.

The enormity of the task of trying to understand such complex behavior can be overwhelming. Where to begin? What aspect or aspects are the important ones to study? Is it possible to understand the whole without a minute study of its parts? If we study the parts, at what level of increasing simplicity do they lose relevance to the whole? These problems confront researchers in all the behavioral sciences, but particularly those disciplines concerned with psychopathology. Certainly research in schizophrenia suffers from them all.

One method used to simplify the problems inherent in studying behavior so complex is to use animal models in which variables acting in the system are more apt to be known and are more amenable to manipulation by the investigator. However, given the complexity of the behavior seen in mental disorders such as schizophrenia, it may be hard to imagine how an animal-model system could be helpful either in furthering our understanding of mental illness or in elucidating the mechanism by which drugs exert their therapeutic effects. In this paper we will attempt to demonstrate the potential usefulness of a specific animal-model system and then briefly point out the limitations of using such a system to study complex human behavior.

While there is increasing evidence that both genes and environment interact to produce such forms of mental disorder as schizophrenia and manic-depressive illness (Rosenthal, 1968; Garmezy, 1972; Kety, 1972), it has not been possible to determine which factors in the external or internal environment interact with what elements in the genotype. However, whatever the relationship between heredity and environment, many people now assume that some organic malfunction must be present in the central nervous system (CNS) to account for at least some of the abnormal behavior observed.

Most recent biochemical theories about possible organic factors in the etiology and pathogenesis of mental illness center around substances that are related to or interact with putative neurotransmitter substances in the brain (Kety and Matthysse, 1972; Kety, 1967). One approach used

by investigators to test their biochemical theories is to look for altered
biochemical processes (e.g., abnormal monoamine metabolites) in
patients with psychiatric disorders. Another approach, which goes hand
in hand with the first, is to develop animal-model systems that permit a
direct study of the neurobiological processes which may underlie
behavioral disorders. In recent years an increasingly important link
between clinical psychiatry and basic neurobiology has developed out of
neuropsychopharmacology. The study of the mechanism of action of
drugs with known clinical effects—both therapeutic and adverse—has
provided the basic researcher with significant clues as to the identity of
neural systems that may be important for the maintenance or disruption
of behavioral processes. Studies of mechanisms of drug action have in
turn led to an intensive investigation of particular neurotransmitter
systems, most notably the monoamines (norepinephrine, NE; dopamine,
DA; and serotonin).

For ethical reasons we are limited in our investigation of drug effects
in humans to the study of easily available body fluids (e.g., cerebrospinal
fluid, blood, and urine). For this reason it becomes necessary to turn to
animals for studies of drug action in the CNS. The model we are
concerned with here is the model provided by the monoamine systems of
the rat brain for elucidating the mechanism of action of drugs. In
particular we will attempt to show how one of these systems, in this case
the DA system, can be used, not only to improve our understanding of
how certain drugs cause behavioral changes in man, but also to predict
the clinical effects of new drugs not yet tested in clinical trials. Although
we will address ourselves solely to the use of the DA system as a test
model, much of what will be said is equally true for the NE and
serotonin systems of the brain.

What characteristics make the monoamine systems of the brain useful
as a model for studying neuropsychopharmacology? In order to answer
this question we have to review some of the developments that have
occurred in the field of histochemistry over the last ten years. Prior to
1964 all anatomical and physiological studies of the CNS were done
without knowledge of the identity of the specific putative neurotransmitter of the pathway under study. In addition many nonmyelinated pathways were unknown since degeneration and staining

techniques were inadequate for their demonstration. Then in 1964 the
Falck-Hillarp fluorescence histochemical technique was applied to brain
tissue, thereby making it possible to map the nonmyelinated NE-, DA-,
and serotonin-containing systems in mammalian brain (Andén et al.,
1964a; Dahlström and Fuxe, 1964). Ungerstedt (1971), using
fluorescence histochemistry combined with lesioning techniques,
mapped the monoamine systems of the rat brain in even greater detail.
Thus, for the first time, neuronal systems in the CNS were both
chemically and anatomically defined. We were provided with a circuit
diagram by which fundamental anatomical, biochemical, and
physiological correlations could be made. The circuit diagram allows for
several types of investigation, including (1) measurement of the
biochemical and physiological changes induced by chemical or
mechanical destruction of specific pathways, and (2) single-unit

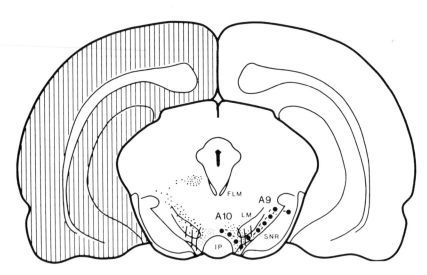

Figure 6.1 A representative transverse section of the rat midbrain at the level of the
interpeduncular nucleus, showing the location of dopamine-containing cell bodies. Black
dots represent dopamine cells in the zona compacta of the substantia nigra (A9) and in the
ventral tegmental area (A10). Abbreviations: FLM, fasciculus longitudinalis medialis; IP,
nucleus interpeduncularis; LM, lemniscus medialis; SNR, substantia nigra, zona reticulata.
From Ungerstedt (1971).

recording from histochemically identified monoaminergic neurons and their postsynaptic (follower) cells for the purpose of investigating physiological function and drug effects at a cellular level. The effect upon unit firing rate induced by various drugs and other substances that alter monoamine turnover can be directly determined by this technique. The histochemical localization of monoamine neuronal perikarya within well-defined nuclei permits a high degree of assurance that recordings in such cases are from bona fide monoamine cells.

One of the catecholamine systems mapped by means of fluorescence histochemical methods was the DA-containing system. It was found that the great majority of DA cells are located in the zona compacta of the substantia nigra and the adjacent midbrain ventral tegmental area (labeled A9 and A10, respectively, by Dahlström and Fuxe; see Figure 6.1). The A9 DA cells project to the caudate nucleus, whereas the A10 DA cells have terminals mainly in the olfactory tubercles and accumbens nucleus (see Figure 6.2). It is important to note that, although the A9 and A10 cell bodies are adjacent to each other in the midbrain, they project to entirely different regions of the brain—the striatal and limbic systems, respectively. It is this precise identification, both anatomical and

DOPAMINE

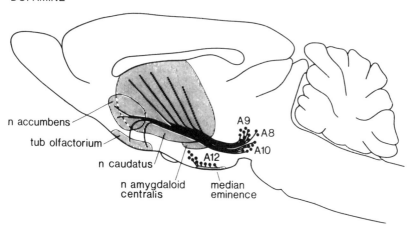

Figure 6.2 Sagittal section of the rat brain showing the projection of dopamine pathways. The dopamine cells in the zona compacta of the substantia nigra (A9) project to the caudate nucleus, whereas the ventral tegmental dopamine cells (A10) project to the nucleus accumbens and olfactory tubercles. Black dots represent cell bodies; stripes indicate terminal areas. From Ungerstedt (1971).

biochemical, that makes the DA system so useful, both in studies of the role of DA in the pathogenesis of disease and as a model in investigations of the central action of certain drugs.

Thanks to the pioneering work of Hornykiewicz we are all aware that the primary anatomical defect in Parkinson's disease is destruction of the dopaminergic neurons in the zona compacta of the substantia nigra. This destruction leads to decreased DA in the neostriatum, which in turn is thought to be responsible for at least some of the symptoms of Parkinson's disease (Hornykiewicz, 1963). Schizophrenic patients treated with antipsychotic drugs often develop symptoms similar to those seen in Parkinson's disease—akinesia, rigidity, and tremor (Klein and Davis, 1969). These side effects, as well as their antipsychotic properties, have been linked by biochemical evidence to an action on the DA system of the brain. This action is thought to be mediated through their ability to block DA receptors.

The first evidence for the central site of action of the antipsychotic phenothiazines came in the 1960s when a group in Sweden headed by Arvid Carlsson examined the effect of these agents on levels of catecholamine metabolites in the CNS. Confirming the earlier findings of Holzer and Hornykiewicz (1959), they failed to show any increase in brain levels of the neurotransmitters themselves after the administration of chlorpromazine (CPZ). However, small doses of CPZ and haloperidol were found to enhance the accumulation of catecholamine metabolites (3-methoxytyramine and normetanephrine) induced by the inhibition of monoamine oxidase (Carlsson and Lindqvist, 1963). The metabolite of DA, homovanillic acid (HVA), was also found to be greatly increased by these drugs (Andén et al., 1964b). More sophisticated biochemical techniques soon followed that allowed various investigators, using a variety of methods, to show that antipsychotic phenothiazines increase DA turnover (Glowinski et al., 1966; Nybäck et al., 1968; Andén et al., 1972). Of equal importance was the fact that phenothiazines lacking antipsychotic efficacy, such as promethazine, had no effect on DA metabolism (Nybäck et al., 1968). Carlsson and Lindqvist (1963) hypothesized that the increase in DA turnover induced by antipsychotic agents may be due, at least in part, to DA-receptor blockade, leading in turn to a compensatory *increase* in DA-cell activity via a neuronal feedback mechanism. In support of this hypothesis both Andén (1971) and Nybäck (1971) have shown that an anatomically intact dopaminergic system must exist for the phenothiazines to cause changes in DA metabolism.

Recently part of Carlsson's hypothesis has been confirmed using single-unit recording techniques. This technique consists of stereotaxically lowering a microelectrode into the brain of an anesthetized or paralyzed animal (in this case an albino rat). The electrical activity of single cells is picked up by the electrode and, through the use of various amplifiers and filters, transferred to an oscilloscope and speaker so that it can be monitored both aurally and visually. At the same time the amplified signal is passed through an analogue computer which then prints out, by means of a recorder, the activity of the cell in the form of a histogram, each line of which represents the integrated rate of firing expressed as spikes per second.

With this technique it has been found that the systemic administration of antipsychotic compounds, including CPZ and haloperidol, does indeed cause an increase in the rate of firing of DA-containing zona compacta (A9) (Bunney et al., 1973a,b; see Figure 6.3). Thus there is evidence that neuroleptics can affect DA metabolism in the striatum through their ability to increase DA-cell activity. Their effect on DA-cell firing rate is thought to be due to an ability to block postsynaptic DA receptors. This blockade, it is suggested, leads to a deficiency of DA at postsynaptic receptors, just as the destruction of DA neurons leads to such a deficiency in Parkinson's disease. It is this line of reasoning that has led investigators to suggest that the antipsychotic drugs may cause their extrapyramidal side effects through the blockade of DA receptors in the neostriatum.

But what about the antipsychotic properties of these drugs? Where is their locus of action? It is tempting to suggest that those cells located in the limbic system that are innervated by A10 DA neurons may be likely candidates. Certainly the limbic system is appealing as a site for such action because of its involvement in emotional expression and behavior, including aspects of sex and aggression (Nauta, 1963; Stevens, 1973). There is biochemical and behavioral evidence both for and against this suggestion. Recently, high levels of dopamine, which are independent of

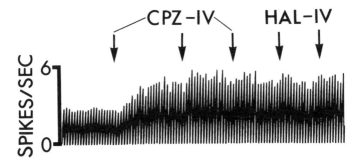

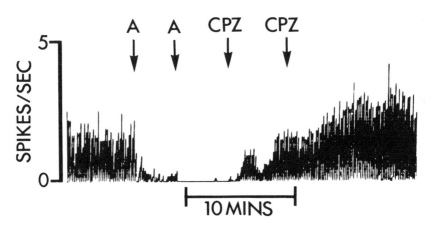

Figure 6.3 Upper tracing: Effect of chlorpromazine (CPZ) on the firing rate of an A9 dopaminergic cell. Intravenous administration of CPZ in a series of small doses (0.5, 0.5, and 1.0 mg/kg) maximally increased firing rate to double its baseline rate. Once a maximal rate of firing was obtained with CPZ, haloperidol (HAL; 0.1 and 0.5 mg/kg) had no further effect, suggesting that these antipsychotic agents act on the same dopamine receptors. From Aghajanian and Bunney (1973). © 1973 by Pergamon Press, Inc. Lower tracing: Antagonism by CPZ of d-amphetamine-induced depression (A) of A9 dopamine-cell activity. Intravenously administered d-amphetamine in a total dose of 0.75 mg/kg stopped the cell completely. After CPZ (0.25 and 0.50 mg/kg) was administered intravenously, cell firing resumed and increased to above baseline levels. From Bunney et al. (1973b). © 1973 by The Williams & Wilkins Co., Baltimore.

known norepinephrine innervation, have been reported to be present in the rat cortex (Thierry et al., 1973). In addition dopamine-containing terminals have been demonstrated in the limbic and frontal cortex by the use of fluorescence histochemical techniques (Hökfelt et al., 1974; Lidbrink et al., 1974). It is quite possible that some of the antipsychotic effects of neuroleptics are mediated through an effect on this system. However, the subcortical limbic system may still be important in mediating neuroleptic antipsychotic properties as there are well-defined connections between this area and the limbic cortex. It must be emphasized, though, that the evidence for the antipsychotic site of action of neuroleptics is not nearly so strong as the evidence for the site of action of neuroleptic-induced extrapyramidal side effects. Nevertheless continued research for the antipsychotic site of action of drugs will lead, it is hoped, to a better understanding of the organic factors contributing to the pathogenesis of schizophrenia.

Another drug whose mechanism of action has been linked to the DA system is d-amphetamine. It produces a paranoid psychosis that many feel is indistinguishable from paranoid schizophrenia and that is rapidly reversed by the antipsychotic agents used in the treatment of schizophrenia (Snyder, 1972). The drug d-amphetamine is thought to stimulate DA receptors indirectly by increasing the release of newly synthesized DA from nerve terminals and blocking its reuptake (Carlsson et al., 1966; Besson et al., 1971a,b). More DA is thus available in the synaptic cleft for the stimulation of DA receptors. Corrodi and coworkers (1967) have hypothesized that increased DA-receptor stimulation would cause a decrease in the DA-cell firing rate mediated by a postsynaptic neuronal feedback pathway. This hypothesis was recently confirmed, again using single-unit recording techniques (Bunney and Aghajanian, 1973). d-Amphetamine in small doses (0.25–1.6 mg/kg) markedly inhibits these cells for prolonged periods of time (Figure 6.4). Interestingly, DA-receptor blockers such as the antipsychotic drugs CPZ and haloperidol reverse the d-amphetamine-induced depression of firing rate (Bunney et al., 1973; see Figure 6.3), thus providing a direct parallel with the interaction of these two drugs in producing and reversing paranoid psychosis in man. The effect of these drugs on DA-cell activity

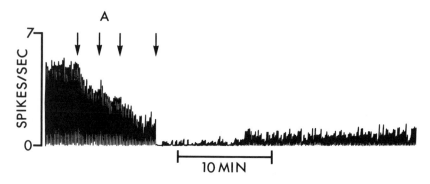

Figure 6.4 Typical effect of d-amphetamine (A) on the activity of dopaminergic cells in the A9 and A10 areas. Serial injections of d-amphetamine (totaling 2.0 mg/kg) progressively depressed cell activity until firing ceased. Recovery was slow—approximately 25% in 30 minutes. From Aghajanian and Bunney (1973). © 1973 by Pergamon Press, Inc.

is selective in that non-DA cells do not respond in a similar manner even at high doses.

In evaluating the significance of the DA neurons as a "model" system, we must first determine whether the ability of CPZ to reverse the d-amphetamine-induced depression of DA-cell firing is a property of all phenothiazines or just ones with antipsychotic properties and/or extrapyramidal side effects. To begin to answer this question promethazine, a drug with little antipsychotic efficacy, few extra-pyramidal side effects (Klein and Davis, 1969), and no effect on DA metabolism (Nybäck et al., 1968), was tested for its ability to reverse the d-amphetamine-induced depression of DA-cell activity in both the A9 and A10 areas. It was found to have no effect (see Figure 6.5) in either area, suggesting that the antipsychotic properties and/or the extrapyramidal side effects of the phenothiazines *are* correlated with the drug's ability to reverse the effects of d-amphetamine. From the data presented so far, however, one cannot distinguish between these possibilities. In order to evaluate this problem further we need to test a phenothiazine which has no antipsychotic efficacy but which does produce extrapyramidal side effects. Such a drug may be mepazine. Using the hypotheses mentioned earlier regarding the site of action of the antipsychotic properties and extrapyramidal side effects of the phenothiazines, we should be able to make some predictions as to the effect mepazine will have on the firing rate of A9 and A10 cells. Since

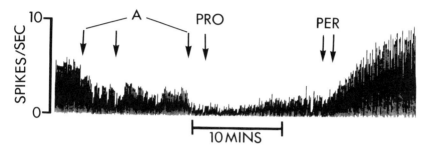

Figure 6.5 Effect of promethazine (PRO) on dopamine-cell activity subsequent to d-amphetamine depression (A). Administration of d-amphetamine (1.25 mg/kg, total dose) depressed unit activity. Promethazine (10 mg/kg i. p.), a phenothiazine lacking antipsychotic efficacy or extrapyramidal side effects, failed to elicit the usual increase in firing rate induced by antipsychotic phenothiazines. The moderate increase in firing rate following promethazine administration is no greater than the spontaneous recovery from amphetamine seen with these cells. However, perphenazine (PER; 0.2 mg/kg, total dose), a clinically active phenothiazine, produced a rapid increase in rate to above baseline levels. From Bunney et al. (1973b). © 1973 by The Williams & Wilkins Co., Baltimore.

mepazine has extrapyramidal side effects and these side effects are thought to be mediated through its action in the nigrostriatal DA system, we predict that mepazine should reverse the d-amphetamine-induced depression of the A9 cell firing rate. But if, as hypothesized, changes in activity of the A10 cells are more closely correlated with the antipsychotic properties of the phenothiazines, such a drug should have no effect on d-amphetamine-induced depression in this cell group. As predicted, when tested for its effect on firing rate, mepazine was found to reverse d-amphetamine-induced depression of DA cells in the A9 group but *not* in the A10 area.

Given these findings, we feel that we may have a model which can be used to differentiate phenothiazines with antipsychotic properties from those lacking clinical efficacy by testing their ability to reverse d-amphetamine-induced depression of A10 dopaminergic neurons. In addition, since mepazine's action is thought to be mediated through its ability to block DA receptors, the above data suggest that there may be important pharmacological differences between DA receptors associated with different DA pathways (e.g., nigrostriatal vs. mesolimbic).

Another obvious question to ask of our model is whether or not it can distinguish an antipsychotic drug with a high incidence of extrapyramidal symptoms from one with a low incidence of these side effects. Since the nigrostriatal DA system is the one most implicated in the pathogenesis of these symptoms, we decided to begin our investigation of this question by comparing the effects on A9 DA-cell activity of two groups of phenothiazines that differ markedly in their incidence of extrapyramidal side effects. We found that antipsychotic drugs with a moderate to high incidence, such as CPZ, perphenazine, trifluoperazine, and haloperidol (Klein and Davis, 1969), increased the activity of A9 cells 50–100% above baseline (see Figure 6.5). In addition, when they reversed d-amphetamine-induced depression of these cells, they always did so to above baseline levels (Figures 6.3, 6.5). However, when antipsychotic drugs with a low incidence of extrapyramidal side effects (e.g., thioridazine and clozapine) were tested, they were found never to increase the firing rate of A9 DA cells to above baseline (Figure 6.6), even when given in doses ten times that needed to reverse d-amphetamine-induced depression. So far, for all phenothiazines tested in our model system, there has been a 100% correlation between their effects on DA-cell activity and their known clinical effects. Thus antipsychotic drugs with a moderate to high incidence of extrapyramidal side effects increase A9 cell activity above baseline rate whether given alone or after d-amphetamine. Conversely antipsychotic drugs with a low incidence of these side effects do not increase A9 cell firing rate.

In summary our data suggest that one might be able to test a new putative antipsychotic drug and predict both its clinical efficacy and the incidence of extrapyramidal side effects by determining its effect on the activity of A9 and A10 cells. In addition this model may provide a means for obtaining the knowledge needed to synthesize drugs with optimal therapeutic efficacy and minimal adverse side effects. Of course the real challenge to our system will come when such a drug is tested, predictions are made, and clinical trials are thereafter begun.

We have discussed here a model system that may help us better understand complex behavior such as schizophrenia through investigations of the way in which certain drugs cause relevant behavioral changes in man. In addition we have tried to demonstrate how this model system may be useful in predicting the clinical effects of new drugs. There are, however, as mentioned in the introduction, problems associated with the use of this kind of model. We are working

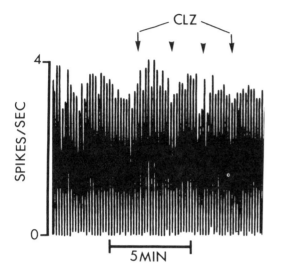

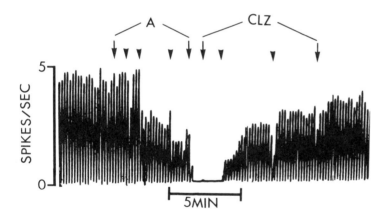

Figure 6.6 Effects of clozapine (CLZ) on the firing rate of dopaminergic neurons in the substantia nigra zona compacta (A9 cell group). Upper Tracing: Clozapine administered intravenously in a total dose of 8 mg/kg had no effect on baseline firing rate. Doses as high as 30 mg/kg i.v. have been tested on other dopamine cells without effect. These results are in marked contrast to those with CPZ, where the average dose needed to increase baseline firing rate 50–100% is approximately 2.0 mg/kg. Lower tracing: Administration of d-amphetamine (A) (1.6 mg/kg i.v.) stopped the firing of this dopamine cell. Clozapine given intravenously in a sequence of doses (1.0, 1.0, 2.0) increased unit activity to 50% of baseline rate. However, an additional 6 mg/kg still did not return activity to baseline levels. CPZ administered after a comparable dose of d-amphetamine would have markedly increased firing rate above baseline in a dose range of 1.5–2.0 mg/kg.

with animals, not humans. Extrapolating from findings in lower animals to man may often be unwarranted, and the difficulties in doing so must always be kept in mind.

In addition, of necessity the biochemist and neuropsychopharma-cologist take a reductionist approach to investigating the etiology and pathogenesis of mental disease. Thus they inherit all the problems inherent in such an approach. They run the risk of myopia, of "not seeing the forest for the trees." Of course the simpler the system studied, the easier it is to know the variables acting on that system and the easier it is to control some of them. However, oversimplicity is also a risk, and one is always plagued with the question of whether or not the changes in the system one is studying are relevant to the complex behavior one is ultimately trying to understand. Although it is certainly legitimate to study either the complex behavior as a whole or elementary units of that behavior, it seems to us doubtful that we will ever know the "whole truth" unless we study both.

References

Aghajanian, G. K., and Bunney, B. S. 1973. Electrophysiological effects of amphetamine on dopaminergic neurons. In S. Snyder and E. Usdin, eds., *Frontiers in catecholamine research.* New York: Pergamon, pp. 957–962.

Andén, N.-E., Carlsson, A., Dahlström, A., Fuxe, K., Hillarp, N.-A., and Larsson, N. 1964a. Demonstration and mapping out of nigro-neostriatal dopamine neurons *Life Sci.* 3:523–530.

Andén, N.-E., Corrodi, H., and Fuxe, K., 1972. Effect of neuroleptic drugs on central catecholamine turnover assessed using tyrosine and dopamine-B-hydroxylase inhibitors. *J. Pharm. Pharmacol.* 24:177–182.

Andén, N.-E., Corrodi, H., Fuxe, K., and Ungerstedt, U. 1971. Importance of nervous impulse flow for the neuroleptic induced increase in amine turnover in central dopamine neurons. *Eur. J. Pharmacol.* 15:193–199.

Andén, N.-E., Roos, B.-E., and Werdinius, B. 1964b. Effects of chlorpromazine, haloperidol and reserpine on the levels of phenolic acids in rabbit corpus striatum. *Life Sci.* 3:149–158.

Besson, M., Cheramy, A., Feltz, P., and Glowinski, J. 1971a. Dopamine: Spontaneous and drug-induced release from the caudate nucleus in the cat. *Brain Res.* 32:407–424.

Besson, M., Cheramy, A., and Glowinski, J. 1971b. Effects of some psychotropic drugs on dopamine synthesis in the rat striatum. *J. Pharmacol. Exp. Ther.* 177:196–205.

Bunney, B. S., Aghajanian, G. K., and Roth, R. H. 1973a. Comparison of effects of

L-DOPA, amphetamine and apomorphine on firing rate of rat dopaminergic neurons. *Nature [New Biol.]* 245:123–125.

Bunney, B. S., Walters, J. R., Roth, R. H., and Aghajanian, G. K. 1973b. Dopaminergic neurons: Effect of antipsychotic drugs and amphetamine on single cell activity. *J. Pharmacol. Exp. Ther.* 185:560–571.

Carlsson, A., Fuxe, K., Hamberger, B., and Lindqvist, M. 1966. Biochemical and histochemical studies on the effects of imipramine-like drugs and (+)-amphetamine on central and peripheral catecholamine neurons. *Acta Physiol. Scand.* 67:481–497.

Carlsson, A., and Lindqvist, M. 1964. Effect on chlorpromazine and haloperidol on formation of 3-methoxytyramine and normetanephrine in mouse brain. *Acta Pharmacol. Toxicol.* 20:140–144.

Corrodi, H., Fuxe, K., and Hökfelt, T. 1967. The effect of some psychoactive drugs on central monoamine neurons. *Eur. J. Pharmacol.* 1:363–368.

Dahlström, A., and Fuxe, K. 1964. Evidence for the existence of monoamine-containing neurons in the central nervous system. *Acta Physiol. Scand. [Suppl.]* 232:1.

Garmezy, N. 1972. Environmental factors in the development of schizophrenia. In Kety and Matthysse (1972), pp. 422–426.

Glowinski, J., Axelrod, J., and Iversen, L. I. 1966. Regional studies of catecholamines in the rat brain. IV. Effects of drugs on the disposition and metabolism of H^3-dopamine. *J. Pharmacol. Exp. Ther.* 153:30–41.

Hökfelt, P., Ljungedahl, A., Fuxe, K., and Johansson, O. 1974. Dopamine nerve terminals in the rat cortex; aspects of the dopamine hypothesis of schizophrenia. *Science* 184:177–179.

Holzer, G., and Hornykiewicz, O. 1959. Uber den Dopamin-(Hydroxytyramin-) Stoffwechsel in Gehirn der Ratte. *Arch. Exp. Pathol. Pharmakol.* 237:27–32.

Hornykiewicz, O. 1963. Die topische Lokalisation und das Verhalten von Noradrenalin und Dopamin-(3-Hydroxytyramin) in der Substantia Nigra des Normalin und Parkinsonkranken. *Wien. Klin. Wochenschr.* 75:309–312.

Kety, S. S. 1967. Current biochemical approaches to schizophrenia. *N. Engl. J. Med.* 276:325–331.

Kety, S. S. 1972. Prospectives for research in schizophrenia—an overview. In Kety and Matthysse (1972), pp. 456–467.

Kety, S. S., and Matthysse, S. 1972. *Prospects for research on schizophrenia.* (*Neurosci. Res. Program Bull.*, vol. 10, no. 4.)

Klein, D. E., and Davis, J. M. 1969. *Diagnosis and drug treatment of psychiatric disorders.* Baltimore: Williams & Wilkins.

Lidbrink, P., Johnsson, G., and Fuxe, K. 1974. Selective reserpine-resistant accumulation of catecholamines in central dopamine neurons after dopa administration. *Brain Res.* 67:439–456.

Nauta, W. J. H. 1963. Central nervous organization and the endocrine motor system. In A. V. Nalbandow, ed., *Advances in neuroendocrinology.* Urbana, Ill.: University of Illinois Press.

Nybäck, H., Borzecki, Z., and Sedvall, G. 1968. Accumulation and disappearance of catecholamines formed from tyrosine-^{14}C in mouse brain: Effect of some psychiatric drugs. *Eur. J. Pharmacol.* 4:395–403.

Nybäck, H., and Sedvall, G. 1971. Effect of nigral lesion of chlorpromazine-induced acceleration of dopamine synthesis from ^{14}C-tyrosine. *J. Pharm. Pharmacol.* 23:322–326.

Rosenthal, D. 1968. The heredity-environment issue in schizophrenia: Summary of the conference and present status of our knowledge. *J. Psychiat. Res.* 6 (Suppl. 1):413–427.

Snyder, S. H. 1972. Catecholamines in the brain as mediators of amphetamine psychosis. *Arch. Gen. Psychiatry* 27:343–351.

Stevens, J. R. 1973. An anatomy of schizophrenia? *Arch. Gen. Psychiatry* 29:177–189.

Thierry, A. M., Stinus, L., Blanc, G., and Glowinski, J. 1973. Some evidence for the existence of dopaminergic neurons in the rat cortex. *Brain Res.* 50:230–234.

Ungerstedt, U. 1971. Stereotaxic mapping of the monoamine pathways in the rat brain. *Acta Physiol. Scand. [Suppl.]* 367:1–48.

7

The Frog's Visual System as a Model for the Study of Selective Attention

David J. Ingle

Introduction

The essence of adaptive behavior for both man and animal involves the ability to select among competing stimuli those most deserving of immediate thought or action, and to choose among alternative responses those most appropriate to the welfare of the organism. As obvious as this might be to any amateur psychologist, the mechanism of "selective attention" to events or actions has not been given due attention in experimental studies of brain function. As a biologist I have been as astonished by this neglect as was the psychologist William James in reviewing his own historical background. In a chapter of his *Principles of Psychology* James invokes our concern for the problem:

Strange to say, so patent a fact as the perpetual presence of selective attention has received hardly any notice from Psychologists of the English empiricist school. . . . The motive of this ignoring of the phenomenon of attention is obvious enough. These writers are bent on showing how the higher faculties of the mind are pure products of "experience," and experience is supposed to be something given. Attention, implying a degree of reactive spontaneity, would seem to break through the circle of pure receptivity which constitutes "experience" and hence must not be spoken of under penalty of interfering with the smoothness of the tale.

But the moment one thinks of the matter, one sees how false a notion of experience that is which would make it tantamount to the mere presence to the senses of an outward order. Millions of items of the outward order are present to my senses which never properly enter into my experience. Why? Because they have no interest for me. My experience is what I agree to attend to. Only those items which I notice shape my mind—without selective interest and emphasis experience is an utter

D. J. Ingle, Neuropsychology Laboratory, McLean Hospital, Belmont, MA, 02178. The author was supported by NIMH Career Scientist Award KO2 13,175, and his research by a grant from the Alfred Sloan Foundation.

chaos. Interest alone gives accent and emphasis, light and shade, background and foreground—intelligible perspective, in a word. It varies in every creature, but without it the consciousness of every creature would be a gray chaotic indiscriminateness, impossible for us even to conceive.

The current emphasis in neuropsychology continues in the empiricist tradition (with some success) in describing mechanisms of stimulus coding and neural activity in systems correlated with fear, aggression, hunger, or sexual drive. It is quite clear that these physiological studies are relevant to theoretical psychiatry since people do manifest pathologies of perception, memory, affect, or impulse-control. Yet, even where no perceptual dysfunction is evident, psychotic patients may show measurable deficits in behaviors that seem to involve "selective attention." (See Chapter 3 for a review of some of the evidence for the importance of attentional deficits in schizophrenia.)

Whatever the relationship of such attentional deficits to the root etiology of mental diseases such as schizophrenia, their manifestation does seem related to the current hypothesis that "biochemical" deficits in functions of the forebrain "limbic system" constitute a fundamental biological predisposition to schizophrenia. The limbic system has numerous fibrous connections with both neocortical and subcortical centers involved in "sensory-motor" or "perceptual" integrations, as well as with lower centers involved in expressions of primary affect. It seems a priori likely that subtle motivational and attentional processes direct the flow of thought and memory at moments when the organism is relatively calm and not in the actual throes of anger, panic, or grief. The many possible modes of influence upon perception, thought, and choice are extremely difficult to tease apart using tools of either the anatomist or the psychologist. The present need to relate new advances in neuro-pharmacology to normal and abnormal behavioral processes can, however, be partially met by focusing physiological and behavioral techniques on a simpler animal system. In the present chapter I shall discuss the feeding system of the common frog as one useful model system in which rudimentary attentional phenomena do seem to be generated by a forebrain complex that is the evolutionary prototype of our own mysterious limbic system.

I have approached the problem of selective attention from a position nearly opposite to that of the clinical psychiatrist, who is concerned with disintegration of the highest levels of personality and adaptive intelligence. As a student of visual behavior I was early led to study the stereotyped behaviors of lower vertebrates as embodiments of basic principles of visual coding and motor selection that could be studied without the complication of such evolutionary refinements as a visual cortex (Ingle, 1968, 1970, 1971, 1973a). In the frog, for example, considerable visual processing is assumed to take place within the retina itself, and indeed a frog retina is structurally more complex than that of a cat or monkey. It seemed likely that the "reflexive" snapping at prey by frogs reflects some direct and simple wiring from the retina into the central nervous system and onto a lower motor center that coordinates the jumping and mouth movements. Indeed Figure 7.1 shows schematically that the frog's optic tectum does both receive retinal fibers

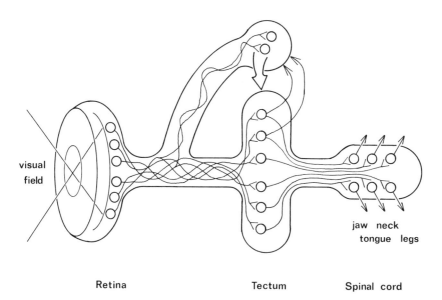

visual field

jaw   neck
tongue legs

Retina   Tectum   Spinal cord

Figure 7.1 A schematic view of the connections of the frog's optic tectum. Each retinal ganglion cell (left) sends its axon through the optic tract to a particular region of tectum (center). Tectal neurons, in turn, send axons to brain-stem and spinal centers (right) where they activate "premotor" systems. Some retinal ganglion cells also project to the visual thalamus (top). Further complexity is introduced into visual analytic processes by reciprocal connections between tectal and thalamic neurons.

and also emit efferent axons that descend to the brain-stem and spinal "motor" centers. Such a straight-through system seems suitable for a neurophysiological and anatomical analysis of both the sensory-filtering and motor-coordination stages of the feeding response. Yet in the course of investigations my own data and that of colleagues invariably revealed motivational and attentional biases that alter the functional state of the retino-tecto-motor system. Consequently I decided to approach the frog as embodying a workable balance between the rigidity of behavior that a physiologist requires and the plasticity of behavior that makes life interesting for a psychologist.

A Model System for Attention

As I have implied, the simplicity of the frog's feeding behavior seemed to offer a major advantage for a physiological analysis of each link in the chain of processes from eye to muscles. However, it is equally important to stress that the behavior to be studied is roughly homologous to the orienting and biting movements of mammalian species who seek to explore or to grasp a newly appearing object. From fish to monkey the retinal projection to the optic tectum plays a major role in alerting the brain to the sudden appearance of small objects to be investigated or the looming of large objects to be avoided (Ingle, 1973a). Thus the neural mechanism that I have studied in the frog has both structural and functional kinship to homologous brain circuits in mammals.

On the other hand the frog's tectum is not "dominated" by major descending projections from neocortex, as is true in cat or monkey. On the behavioral side the feeding behavior of the frog is less obviously altered by learning than is that of a mammal. The visually guided feeding system of the frog therefore reveals a basic *mode* of action that appears in mammals as well, but the *context* determining when that action is released is much more complex among mammals. If the experimenter's aim is to understand how a monkey or a man views his particular decisions, our bug-catching model will not get us very far. However, if we seek to unravel fundamental neural mechanisms by which motivational states influence the operations of sensorimotor systems, then the frog's uncomplicated view of life can prove most refreshing.

A second consideration in choosing a model system for analysis of attention is strictly technical: in order to understand how an organism "switches in" a response to one stimulus at the expense of another, we must know how the two stimuli differ in critical attributes and how these attributes are coded within the sensory systems. It is also necessary to specify which stimulus has gained attention at a particular moment in order to create an unambiguous context for physiological monitoring of relevant brain circuits. However, for mammals, we simply do not know how information about the color or shape of objects is encoded beyond the early filtering mechanisms described in visual cortex. Furthermore, in psychological studies (whether in rat or man), the operation of attention is inferred from behavioral trends averaged over many trials and can seldom be specified on any given stimulus presentation, as the physiologist would wish.

For these reasons I have studied the processes by which the frog attends to objects on the basis of *spatial* location. We know, of course, that the visual system is topographically organized and that neurons at each level of processing (retina, thalamus, tectum, cortex) respond to visual events within a restricted region of the visual field. It seems possible that readiness to respond to events in one region of space (or to ignore them) is dependent upon prior facilitative or inhibitive effects in a selected region of one or more central relay stations.

At all levels of vertebrate phylogeny the optic tectum (or the superior colliculus in mammals) participates in the orientation of eyes, head, or body toward visual stimuli of "interest" to the particular organism. In this sense the act of making a rapid orientation toward a suddenly moved object in order to "evaluate" the prospects for approach or flight is "functionally equivalent" from fish to man and involves the coordination of homologous sensory and motor organs (retina, tectum, spinal cord, neck and eye muscles). Some of the similarities and differences in visual-coding mechanisms and motor patterns among vertebrate groups have been reviewed in detail (Ingle, 1973a; Ingle and Sprague, 1975). For the present discussion the important function of the retinotectal system is the selection of a *single* visual target to guide the response, whether it be foveation in a monkey or a tongue flick in a frog. Both frogs and monkeys can be said to attend *selectively* to visual objects since they usually respond to but one of several potentially equipotent stimuli in simultaneous view (Ingle, 1973b). It is important for our definition of selective attention that circumstances can easily bias the animal to respond at other times to a different object. Of course attachments to particular objects can reflect prior learning, and we shall exclude this type of response bias from our consideration of short-term attentional processes.

The optic projections of all vertebrate classes include four apparently homologous regions (dorsal thalamus, pretectum, tectum, and accessory optic tract), each of which appears to participate in a specialized mode of visual processing. The tecta of all species receive axons from motion-sensitive retinal or cortical cells, and tectal neurons accordingly seem to be specialized for noticing sudden motions of relatively small objects within localized regions of the visual field. Some tectal neurons send efferent axons into tegmental, pontine, and spinal centers which participate in the control of body, head, or eye movements. In the frog, at least, some efferent cells apparently contact both retinal axons and spinal neurons (Szekely, 1973). However, frogs do not usually turn or snap at every small moving stimulus. Their behavior depends upon both the nature of the particular stimulus and the course of prior events. The tectum, then, is an active "filter" that is modulated by other brain structures. In mammals prominent corticotectal pathways bias or even dominate the response characteristics of tectal neurons. Yet the frog tectum operates without direct communication from the telencephalon, and, in fact, the frog has no identifiable homologue of neocortex to complicate his life. For these reasons we assume that the attentional biases operating upon the frog's tectum are more easily isolated than those operating in mammals.

Basic Neurobehavioral Units in the Frog's Feeding Behavior
In order to isolate the operations of the attentional mechanism we must first identify the basic components of the sensorimotor system in question. The germinal studies of Lettvin and coworkers (1961) called attention to the filtering properties of so-called bug-detector units in the frog's retina. These units are optimally sensitive to small dark objects moving within the 3–5° receptive fields. Their axon terminals are recorded in the superficial region of the tectal neuropil, where they come

into synaptic contact with dendrites from deeper cell laminae (Szekely, 1973). The first cell lamina (Figure 7.2) contains pear-shaped neurons that are sensitive to small moving stimuli rather than to changes of illumination or the motion of very large stimuli. These cells rapidly habituate to repeated motion of objects within their receptive fields and have therefore been designated by Lettvin and coworkers (1961) as "newness neurons."

These neurons are probably not the efferent neurons that discharge directly into "motor" centers. For one thing such long axons are more likely to arise from larger pyramidal cells located in still deeper tectal laminae. Furthermore many newness neurons have receptive fields

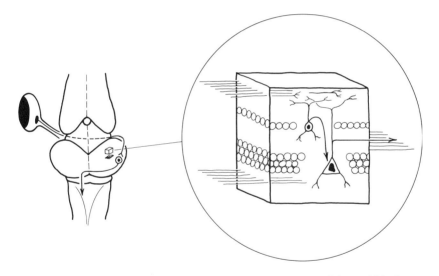

Figure 7.2 The author's hypothetical view of the essential visuomotor linkage within the frog's optic tectum. In cross section, a heavy cellular lamina dominates in the deeper tectum, while a thinner cell lamina is evident more superficially. Large pyramidal neurons in the deep lamina are thought to provide efferent axons to lower premotor structures whose activity generates stereotyped feeding or avoidance movements. Neurons in the superficial lamina include the rapidly habituating "newness cells" whose activity appears to be related to the elicitation of feeding behavior by small moving objects. The present hypothesis utilizes the descending intrinsic axons (seen in Golgi-stained material) as links by which newness neurons facilitate tectal efferent neurons. This input would enhance the probability that the frog will turn or snap at the stimulus. But—according to this model—moderate discharge of newness neurons (as in the frog paralyzed for recording) would not trigger the efferent neurons. From Ingle (1973a). Reprinted with permission of S. Karger AG, Basel.

located 10–20° away from the retinotopic locus of the retinal axon terminals that are recorded in the same vertical penetration. The discharge of these "displaced" neurons would not guide the frog to the appropriate target were they directly coupled to the motor system. It is our best current guess that newness neurons help to focus the frog's attention on relevant prey stimuli and that, when their activity is high, they facilitate the action of the "efferent-command" neurons that initiate the orienting movement.

The fact that newness neurons habituate rapidly helps to explain the behavioral habituation found in studies of prey-catching behavior (Ewert, 1970; Ewert and Ingle, 1971). When a prey-like object is moved several times within a particular region of the visual field, a frog or toad tends to lose interest in further movements within that particular locus, but will still respond promptly to stimuli appearing more than 30° distant from that region (Eikmanns, 1955; Ewert and Ingle, 1971). I have found that as few as four or five repeated movements of a small worm-like object in one lateral monocular field are sufficient to induce frogs to snap at the opposite member of a symmetrical, synchronously moved pair of stimuli (Ingle, 1973c). After a series of four habituating motions separated by five seconds, one must wait at least twenty seconds before this localized habituation tendency decays. The more prolonged the stimulation, the longer the "selective inattention" lasts. Individual tectal neurons usually require fifteen to thirty seconds to recover from even a single stimulation trial (Lettvin et al., 1961; Ingle, 1973d), so that the neurobehavioral correlations are roughly appropriate.

The Neural Mechanism of Habituation in the Optic Tectum
It is clear from studies of Thompson (see Chapter 9) that neural habituation can occur within a monosynaptic circuit and does not necessarily require interneuronal inhibitory feedback processes. In the frog tectum it is possible that optic-fiber terminals have a self-limiting mechanism that lasts many seconds, due either to transmitter depletion or to inhibition of further transmitter release, as suggested by Horn (1967). However, two facts appear to refute that hypothesis as a major explanation of newness-neuron or behavioral habituation in the frog. First, habituation can be most easily achieved by moving very large

black stimuli within one monocular field and testing with small prey-like stimuli. Yet the class-2 "bug-detector" retinal axons are but weakly activated by large stimuli, and newness neurons are also more responsive to small objects. Second, habituation to moving prey is abolished after large lesions are made in the contralateral posterior thalamic region (Ewert, 1970).

The disinhibition syndrome produced by such thalamic lesions deserves special comment since it provides a major clue as to the physiology of attentional mechanisms in anuran amphibians. The effective lesion to produce this unique syndrome is either a knife cut that severs tectum from thalamus or destruction of the posterolateral cell region. As soon as frogs or toads recover from anesthesia, they show an abnormal tendency to orient toward every moving object. Instead of preferring as prey objects of about 5° visual angle (when three inches from the eye), toads respond optimally to stimuli of up to 30°—a size that they would normally avoid. Thus a selective preference for small objects is abolished as well as the ability to ignore stimuli that have been presented recently.

I have examined Ewert's hypothesis that posterior thalamic lesions eliminate or interrupt an inhibitory pathway from thalamus that directly modulates the optic tectum. Taking frogs with disinhibited feeding behavior, I recorded newness neurons in the first tectal cell lamina, measuring both receptive-field size and habituation rate (Ingle, 1973d). In disinhibited frogs most neurons had receptive fields ranging from 20° to 30°, roughly twice the size of the fields in normal frogs. Furthermore the habituation rate was much reduced in the lesioned frogs and did not exceed the level of adaptation already found in the retinofugal class-2 fiber terminals (Figure 7.3) that must activate the neurons. Apparently the newness neurons in the disinhibited animal could not ignore their axodendritic input and faithfully followed the retinal discharge. When the lesion had produced only a partial disinhibition effect (e.g., only for stimuli in the rostral visual field of one eye), we found hyperexcitable tectal neurons only in the corresponding region of tectum.

Subsequent studies using the Fink-Heimer stain for degenerating axon terminals showed that the posterolateral cell region of the posterior thalamus does indeed give rise to a prominent projection in the optic

Class 1 or 2

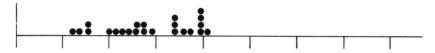

Normal cells

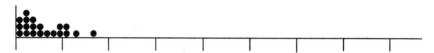

Tectal cells after PT lesion

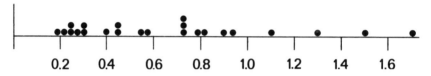

| 0.2 | 0.4 | 0.6 | 0.8 | 1.0 | 1.2 | 1.4 | 1.6 |

Figure 7.3 Overview of data obtained from recording experiments with normal or with surgically "disinhibited" frogs. The latter group showed excessive nonhabituating prey-catching behavior toward moving objects. Each black circle represents the data of a particular tectal multiple-cell group (that is, three to five units), where eight responses to spot motion were recorded. The sum of four responses after 10-second recovery intervals was divided by the sum of four intervening responses obtained after 60-second recovery intervals to give the "habituation ratio" (that is, the number of spikes at 10-second intervals per 60 seconds) for each unit population. While afferent inputs from the eye (class 1 or 2 fibers) show significant adaptation after a 10-second recovery, the normal postsynaptic cells show a much greater decrement (habituation). The second process does not appear after appropriate pretectal lesions and, therefore, is not intrinsic to the tectum. From Ingle (1973d). © 1973 by the American Association for the Advancement of Science.

tectum (Trachtenberg and Ingle, 1974). These axons terminate in both superficial neuropil and in deeper cell laminae. Thus thalamic axons might either modulate axodendritic flow superficially or inhibit cell bodies in deeper laminae.

Whatever the exact synaptic mechanism, studies using topical application of strychnine have produced a tectal-neuron disinhibition in frogs that is qualitatively similar to that obtained via thalamic lesions (Stevens, 1973). Unpublished data from our laboratory also indicate that localized strychnine treatment produces foci of disinhibition such that any moving object within an area as small as 30–40° can elicit a turn or snap. This suggests that the thalamotectal modulation depends upon a cholinergic inhibitory synapse.

The notion that activation of the thalamotectal inhibitory system results in a short-term suppression of prey-catching tendencies is in line with recording data from the posterolateral cell region (Ewert, 1971; Brown and Ingle, 1973). Most of the isolated neurons in this region of thalamus respond much better to large than to small objects and more strongly via the contralateral than via the ipsilateral eye. Inhibition of feeding is best induced by large objects and can be lateralized to the contralateral side. An additional property of many posterior thalamic units is their prolonged afterdischarge elicited by a black object moving briefly into and out of view. The ten- to twenty-second poststimulus burst of some presumably inhibitory neurons is in rough agreement with the interval of poststimulus suppression seen among many tectal neurons. This problem is in need of quantitative study since the matching of time constants between thalamic and tectal processes is critical to this hypothesis.

The anatomical, physiological, and psychosurgical data that I have briefly reviewed indicate that a subset of posterior thalamic neurons sends inhibitory input directly to the optic tectum, and by this mechanism modulates the intensity and temporal course of feeding behavior toward moving visual stimuli. We might further ask how such visually responsive cells are themselves activated. At first thought the retinal projection into the posterior thalamic neuropil (Szekely, 1973) seems to be a likely route for direct excitation of the postsynaptic cells of this region. In a recent study (Brown and Ingle, 1973), however, we found that the wide-field neurons of the posterior thalamus (which respond best to large objects and often given an afterdischarge to briefly presented objects) derive most or all of their input from the optic tectum. If the ipsilateral tectum is removed, no wide-field contralateral visual activation is present through the opposite eye. If small, focal, tectal lesions are made, each wide-field posterior thalamic neuron has a "scotoma" in the appropriate part of its visual field. In tectum-lesioned frogs many small-field neurons remain, and these presumably do receive direct retinal input. In summary it appears that neurons of the posterolateral cell complex are part of a feedback loop that originates in the tectum itself. Besides the "newness neurons," which are generally selective for small moving objects, the tectum harbors many neurons that respond well to large black stimuli, including the turning off of room lights. This subset of tectal neurons is the best candidate for projection forward into posterior thalamus.

Of course the posterior thalamic neurons are probably themselves influenced by the activity of brain circuits other than the optic tectum. Ewert (1971) finds many of them activated by tactile input in the toad, and some of these can change their threshold to visual stimulation for many seconds after the skin has been touched. Ewert (1970) also reports that the feeding behavior of toads can be strikingly altered by the presentation of familiar prey odor (from crushed mealworms), so that the olfactory system must also modulate visual-motor functions in some fashion. It is interesting in this regard to note that Scalia (1972) has traced the accessory olfactory tract of the frog into the amygdala region of the telencephalon, while Halpern (1972) has traced projections from that region into the posterolateral cell group of the thalamus. These neural circuits could mediate excitatory effects of odor on the toad's readiness to feed by reducing activity of posterior thalamic neurons and so releasing tectal neurons from the usual restraint. As a broad hypothesis my suggestion that frog telencephalon facilitates rather than initiates action sequences is similar to that of Aronson and Kaplan (1968), who have reviewed possible functions of the fish forebrain.

The postulation of a telencephalic-diencephalic control loop (see Figure 7.4) that modulates the diencephalic-mesencephalic feeding/avoidance systems may help us to interpret certain paradoxical effects of "depressant" agents, such as ethanol, which at low doses actually facilitate some behaviors. For example, Ryback (1969) observed that the maze-learning ability of goldfish is enhanced by a few hours' swimming within a 400 mg% solution but is depressed by a 650 mg% dose. More recently I have observed that moderate alcohol intoxication in frogs strikingly increases the frequency of avoidance responses to an overhead rotating object (a simulated "predator"), while a higher dose will abolish the same avoidance behavior.

This bimodal effect of ethanol on a simple behavior might be explained by the hypothesis that a lower alcohol dose reduces the

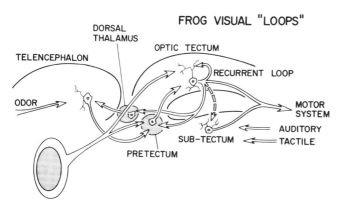

Figure 7.4 A schematic overview of some connections among visual centers in the frog. Visual "loops" of three sizes are suggested. First, an intrinsic loop within the optic tectum, based upon ascending recurrent axons from deeper cell layers. Second, tectofugal connections to the caudal half of the dorsal thalamus terminate near neurons which give rise to a thalamotectal pathway. Third, pathways pass both directions between thalamus and telencephalon, although not apparently connecting the same reciprocal cell masses. Thus output from some tectal neurons may initiate "feedback" chains of varying lengths which themselves modulate tectal activity.

activity of the telencephalic neurons that inhibit posterior thalamic cells (thus releasing avoidance behavior) while higher alcohol treatment directly depresses the thalamotectal substrate of the jumping response. In support of this idea it should be noted that goldfish suffering ablation of telencephalon can show a paradoxically faster acquisition rate in a Y maze (Ingle, 1965) and that toads with most of the telencephalon removed show signs of hyperavoidance behavior (Ewert, 1970).

Animal Models of Attention: An Analysis of Amphetamine Effects
One current model of the schizophrenic type of psychosis is that produced in man by the chronic administration of amphetamine (Ellinwood, 1968; Snyder, 1972). In mammalian species, including rat, cat, and monkey, a set of symptoms develop during chronic amphetamine treatment that strikingly resembles some stereotypic human behaviors related to amphetamine intoxication. In early treatment a hyperattentive state with persistent "investigative" behavior is seen in which small objects or slight sounds repeatedly gain attention or are pursued for inspection. Orientation toward events in the

peripheral fields is particularly enhanced. Habituation to familiar sensations (sound, odors, skin prickliness) fails, and the subject cannot ignore the many insignificant bombardments of his sensorium. Straschill and Hoffman (1969) report that neurons in the cat optic tectum are dishabituated by intravenous doses of amphetamine. Yet direct iontophoretic application of norepinephrine or dopamine only depresses individual tectal cells in their response to visual stimuli (Straschill and Perwein, 1971), suggesting that the dishabituation of tectal neurons that follows intravenous injections is mediated by extrinsic "modulators" of tectal activity. Sprague and coworkers (1966) noticed that some tectal cells suddenly become more sensitive to moving stimuli during spontaneous occurrence of high-frequency "arousal" signs in the cortical EEG. Chi and Flynn (1968) report that visually evoked potentials in the cat optic tectum can be augmented by concurrent hypothalamic stimulation, an effect which might also reflect intensification of corticotectal control.

Yet, during repeated doses of amphetamine, the characteristic approach behaviors of cats or monkeys toward various stimuli progressively change into hyperfearful reactions to various events. A cat may react with terror to its own shadow, or a human subject may express continual fear of being assailed from behind. In some way continued hyperstimulation of a neural subsystem results in the release of opposing types of behavior (hyperavoidance) without decreasing the "arousal" level. This "progressive-disease" model may be used to investigate two primary questions: (1) Where in the brain does amphetamine first offset the balance of attentional and motivational mechanisms? (2) How do compensatory mechanisms operate which may themselves bring forth the psychotic symptoms? Does overstimulation of the approach system (seen as hyperexploration) either fatigue this system or augment negative feedback mechanisms that then overwhelm the approach mechanism? Telencephalic-diencephalic and diencephalic-mesencephalic feedback loops offer a possible substrate for such hypothetical compensatory phenomena.

Reviewing the literature on amphetamine-induced stereotypies in mammalian behavior brings to mind the overtly similar psychopathology sometimes seen in toads that have recovered from the disinhibition syndrome induced by knife cuts through the posterior thalamus. After a few weeks toads that once had excessive prey-catching activity may show visual-avoidance activity again, perhaps because severed thalamotectal axons are capable of regeneration. Yet some toads show excessive avoidance tendencies such that they duck or scramble away if the experimenter approaches to within several feet (unlike normal toads who are habituated to humans and readily feed from one's hand). They even demonstrate "paranoid" behavior to each other, ducking as a neighbor toad approaches in pursuit of a worm.

Two types of explanation seem plausible. First, recovery of tectothalamic integration following axonal regeneration might simply unmask the effects of permanent damage to the thalamic fibers or cells that inhibit avoidance behavior. Indeed we have several times seen the "hyperavoidance" syndrome following relatively small lesions just rostral to the posterior thalamus. Second, hyperstimulation of prey catching might itself set in motion a feedback process that *reduces* telencephalic inhibition of posterior thalamic neurons. An analogous feedback mechanism was discussed in Chapter 6, where it was postulated that activation of dopamine receptors in telencephalon induces feedback inhibition of mesencephalic or diencephalic neurons. The idea that changes in efferent control by telencephalic projections might underlie "adaptation" to the effects of caudal thalamic lesions is made the more plausible by the observations of Ewert (personal communication) that signs of disinhibited prey catching can be restored—even after normalization—by ablation of most of the telencephalon.

Studies on the effect of amphetamine on the motivational state of lower vertebrates would be interesting, in light of the popular hypothesis (Snyder, 1972) that amphetamine-induced stereotypies may reflect hyperstimulation of dopamine (DA) receptors in either the basal forebrain region or the corpus striatum. Fog et al. (1970) report that amphetamine-induced stereotypies are abolished by large striatum lesions in the rat, but the situation is complicated by the failure of McKenzie (1972) to observe effects of striatal damage on similar stereotyped behavior produced by injections of apomorphine. However, McKenzie did find abolition of these pathological manifestations by lesions within the olfactory tubercle—another region rich in DA terminals. However, Parent (1973) finds no comparable DA-rich area in the frog's striatum, although some fluorescence appears in the basal forebrain and hypothalamus. Our unpublished observations indicate that amphetamine injections at doses ranging from 1 to 10 mg/kg do not produce stereotyped behaviors in frogs. This failure may be related to the relatively sparse green fluorescence patterns seen in frogs by Parent, compared with reptiles or with mammals. However, A. Campbell—in our laboratory—has recently observed that doses of amphetamine as low as 3 mg/kg elicit well-defined stereotypic feeding patterns in the goldfish. In this species DA concentrations in whole brain appear comparable to those in mammals (Shashoua, 1973), but no descriptions of telencephalic fluorescence patterns have yet appeared. Since goldfish with telencephalon ablated show normal feeding and avoidance behaviors, it would be important to examine their responses to amphetamine (or to apomorphine). If the direct effect of amphetamine upon hypothalamic NE or DA neurons in fishes is to initiate stereotyped feeding, one would be the more inclined to explore homologous effects in mammalian hypothalamus. Those experiments may be neglected due to the apparent adequacy of the striatal-DA hypothesis. Such provocation is, of course, a major function of a good model system.

Concluding Remarks

The experiments that I have summarized lead to the hypothesis that collaboration between diencephalic and mesencephalic visual centers is required both for selective feeding behavior and for adaptive shifts in the motivational control of feeding. Other facts have led to the proposal that telencephalic circuits impose more subtle modulating effects upon primary emotional expression in frogs and fishes, including homeostatic response to brain injury or to drug effects. In order to pursue (1) pharmacological hypotheses of drug action or (2) theories of genetic dysfunction of emotional behavior, the localization of critical synaptic junctions within telencephalic and diencephalic control systems will be necessary. Furthermore a general understanding of the behavioral outputs of those neural "loops" that integrate higher and lower brain centers is required for predicting the effects of localized neurotransmitter dysfunction. The relative simplicity of these loops in the brains of fishes or frogs seems to be a compelling argument for the use of these species as "model systems." The behavioral dysfunctions already observed in these animals following brain lesions and drug treatments seem sufficiently similar to those seen among mammals to justify the "relevance" requirement of a good model system. It is to be hoped that psychiatrists will follow up their recent discovery that human behavior has firm roots in the anthropoid past with further excursions into the ethological literature, where sagas of love and hate have been written for the fishes as well.

References

Aronson, L. R., and Kaplan, H. 1968. Function of the teleostean forebrain. In D. Ingle, ed., *The central nervous system and fish behavior*. Chicago: University of Chicago Press.

Brown, W., and Ingle, D. 1973. Receptive field changes produced in frog thalamic units by lesions of the optic tectum. *Brain Res.* 59:405–409.

Chi, C. C., and Flynn, J. P. 1968. The effects of hypothalamic and reticular stimulation on evoked responses in the visual system of the cat. *Electroencephalogr. Clin. Neurophysiol.* 24:343–356.

Eikmanns, V. K.-H. 1955. Verhaltensphysiologische Untersuchungen über den Beutefang und das Bewegungssehen der Erdkröte *(Bufo bufo* L.). *Z. Tierpsychol.* 12:229–253.

Ellinwood, E. H. 1968. Amphetamine psychosis II. Theoretical implications. *Int. J. Neuropsychiatry* 4:45–54.

Ewert, J. P. 1970. Neural mechanisms of prey-catching and avoidance behavior in the toad *(Bufo bufo* L.). *Brain Behav. Evol.* 3:36–56.

Ewert, J. P. 1971. Single unit responses of the toad's *(Bufo americanus)* caudal thalamus to visual objects. *Z. Vergl. Physiol.* 74:81–102.

Ewert, J. P., and Ingle, D. 1971. Excitatory effects following habituation of prey-catching activity in frogs and toads. *J. Comp. Physiol. Psychol.* 77:369–374.

Fog, R., Randrup, A., and Pakkenberg, H. 1970. Lesions in corpus striatum and cortex of rat brains and the effect on pharmacologically induced stereotyped, aggressive and cataleptic behavior. *Psychopharmacol.* 18:346–356.

Halpern, M. 1972. Some connections at the telencephalon of the frog *(Rana pipiens)*. An experimental study. *Brain Behav. Evol.* 6:42–68.

Horn, G. 1967. Neuronal mechanisms of habituation. *Nature* 215:707–711.

Ingle, D. 1965. Behavioral effects of forebrain lesions in goldfish. *Proc. Am. Psychol. Assoc.* 1:143.

Ingle, D. 1968. Visual releasers of prey catching behavior in frogs and toads. *Brain Behav. Evol.* 1:500–518.

Ingle, D. 1970. Visuomotor functions of the frog optic tectum. *Brain Behav. Evol.* 3:57–71.

Ingle, D. 1971. Prey catching behavior of Anurans toward moving and stationary objects. *Vision Res.* [Suppl. 3], pp. 447–456.

Ingle, D. 1973a. Evolutionary perspectives on the function of the optic tectum. *Brain Behav. Evol.* 8:211–237.

Ingle, D. 1973b. Selective choice between double prey objects by frogs. *Brain Behav. Evol.* 7:127–144.

Ingle, D. 1973c. Reduction of habituation of prey catching by alcohol intoxication in the frog. *Brain Behav. Biol.* 8:123–129.

Ingle, D. 1973d. Disinhibition of tectal neurons by pretectal lesions in the frog. *Science* 180:422–424.

Ingle, D., and Sprague, J. 1975. Sensorimotor functions of the optic tectum. *Neurosci. Res. Program Bull.* (in press).

James, W. 1950. *Principles of psychology.* New York: Dover (reprint of 1890 edition), vol. 1, chap. 11.

Kicliter, E. 1973. An anatomical connection between the anterior thalamus and the telencephalon in the frog. *Society for Neuroscience Third Annual Meeting* (abstract).

Lettvin, J. Y., Maturana, H. R., McCulloch, W. S., and Pitts, W. H. 1961. Two remarks on the visual system of the frog. In W. A. Rosenblith, ed., *Sensory communication.* Cambridge, Mass.: The MIT Press.

McKenzie, G. M. 1972. Role of the tuberculum olfactorium in stereotyped behavior induced by apomorphine in the rat. *Psychopharmacologia* 23:212–219.

Parent, A. 1973. Distribution of monoamine-containing neurons in the brain stem of the frog, *Rana temporaria. J. Morphol.* 139:67–78.

Ryback, R. S. 1969. Effect of ethanol, bourbon and various ethanol levels on Y-maze learning in the goldfish. *Psychopharmacologia* 14:305–314.

Scalia, F. 1972. The projection of the accessory olfactory bulb in the frog. *Brain Res.* 36:409–411.

Shashoua, V. E. 1974. Biogenic amine effects on brain metabolism. *Brain Res.* (in press).

Snyder, S. H. 1972. Catacholamines in the brain as mediators of amphetamine psychosis. *Arch. Gen. Psychiatry* 27:169–179.

Sprague, J. M., Marchiafava, P. L., and Rizzolati, G. 1968. Unit responses to visual stimuli in the superior colliculus of the unanesthetized mis-pontine cat. *Arch. Ital. Biol.* 106:169–193.

Stevens, R. J. 1973. A cholinergic inhibitory system in the frog optic tectum: Its role in visual electrical responses in feeding behavior. *Brain Res.* 49:309–321.

Straschill, M., and Hoffman. 1969. Effect of d-amphetamine on the activity of single neurons of the cat's optic tectum. *Experientia* 52:373.

Straschill, M., and Perwein, J. 1971. Effect of iontophoretically applied biogenetic amines and of cholinomimetic substances upon the activity of neurons in the superior colliculus and mesencephalic reticular formation of the cat. *Pflügers Arch.* 324:43–55.

Szekely, G. 1973. Anatomy and synaptology of the optic tectum. In *Handbook of sensory physiology.* Heidelberg: Springer-Verlag, vol. 7, part 3B, pp. 1–26.

Trachtenberg, M. C., and Ingle, D. 1974. Thalamo-tectal projections in the frog. *Brain Res.* 79:419–430.

8
Processes Controlling Aggressive Behavior in Cichlid Fish

Walter Heiligenberg

Introduction

Aggression and violence in man are of great concern to many psychiatrists. Different and often rather dogmatic views have been expressed about the causation of human aggression (Lorenz, 1963; Scott, 1968, 1971) and different remedies have been offered accordingly. Whereas some scientists (exemplified by Lorenz) stress the adaptive biological significance of aggressive behavior in animals, including man, and consider patterns of aggression to be largely genetically determined, others (including most American psychologists) tend to interpret aggression in man as an environmental and educational consequence rather than as part of his genetic heritage. This controversy largely rests upon the loose and inaccurate use of the word aggression, which covers both the existence of aggressive behavioral patterns and the organism's motivation to perform them. Whereas most scientists accept the proposition that neurological coordinating mechanisms controlling certain behavioral patterns are built-in features of the animal organism, no such general agreement would be found with respect to the motivation of aggressive behavior.

Animal experiments are commonly used in physiology to study mechanisms which for technical or ethical reasons are difficult to approach in humans. In addition complex physiological systems are often found in simpler version among lower animals and may thus be easier to study. The many similarities between human and animal aggression support the notion of common features governing its causation. Studies on animal aggression may therefore shed light on the similar but far more complex phenomena found in man and thus help to

W. Heiligenberg, Scripps Institution of Oceanography, University of California at San Diego, La Jolla, CA, 92037.

resolve some present controversies in human psychology. Animal-model systems of sufficient simplicity thus are needed to investigate certain key problem areas: (1) the genetic and environmental sources of aggression; (2) the role of stimuli in arousing or inhibiting aggression; (3) the physiological consequences of dominance and inferiority; and (4) possible mechanisms to divert aggressive tendencies into "harmless" activities.

A major obstacle in this approach is the diversity of aggressive behaviors found in the animal kingdom. Certain patterns of behavior may serve to space out ecological competitors, mostly members of the same species, while different patterns may be employed in predator-prey interactions (Eibl-Eibesfeldt, 1970). Thus we make a distinction between *intra*specific and *inter*specific aggression. In addition aggressive behavior may fulfill different functions for different species (e.g., securing feeding resources in one species and defending breeding sites in another). Because of this functional diversity different physiological mechanisms may be found to control aggression in different species of animals (Rasa, 1970; Courchesne and Barlow, 1971; Heiligenberg and Kramer, 1972; Frank, 1973). Therefore, since aggression is not a unitary phenomenon, it seems impossible to arrive at a monistic principle covering all forms of aggression in all species of animals. Particular caution should guide attempts to generalize across species.

To investigate mechanisms underlying aggressive behavior one would start with "lower" animals in the hope that their behavior is of a more stereotyped nature and less contaminated by individual experience. This should simplify experimental procedures and make a quantitative analysis easier. This paper will review some quantitative studies on aggression linked to territorial behavior in cichlid fish.

General Features of Cichlid Behavior
Cichlids are a large family of fish found in Africa and South America. Their most striking feature is a highly developed social behavior. Various forms of family and group organization are found in different genera of these animals, with a large variety of behavioral patterns accompanying such activities as territorial defense, pair formation, building and

preparation of breeding sites, and spawning and raising of larvae and young fish.

Young cichlids commonly grow up in schools. As single males reach sexual maturity, they tend to settle down in territories and to attack intruders. Whereas small opponents are chased away and occasionally bitten, large opponents are attacked more hesitantly. Both animals may go through a series of mutual displays by intensifying particular color patterns and presenting body and fin postures that enlarge their overall contours. Unless one combatant withdraws from this encounter, a vigorous fight may ensue in which both animals bite and ram each other until one of them flees from the territory. Such fights may last for hours and lead to considerable injuries and exhaustion. Females ready to spawn or to settle down in a male's territory perform particular behavioral patterns that make attacks by the resident male less likely.

A territorial male will attack adult conspecific males most vigorously, whereas smaller intruders are only chased occasionally. Not only do adult conspecific males elicit attacks more frequently, they also appear to raise a general readiness to attack in a resident male. This can be most easily demonstrated by presenting a conspecific rival for several seconds behind a glass partition. Even if no overt fighting is elicited during this short confrontation, the resident male will thereafter attack the other fish in its environment more frequently than it would have without this stimulation. This suggests that the readiness to attack other fish may, at least to some extent, be controlled by specific stimuli. This phenomenon will be investigated in the following sections.

Experimental Procedures

The readiness in an animal to attack may be measured by the frequency of attacks elicited by a standardized test stimulus. When a territorial male cichlid is living in a large communal tank with both adult conspecifics and small juveniles available for attacking, the rates of attacks directed against these two types of target are found to be proportional. When, for example, the per-half-hour rate of attacks against adults increases by a certain factor, approximately the same increase will be noted in the rate of attacks against juveniles (Leong, 1969). The fact that the rates of attacks directed against these two types of target are highly positively correlated suggests that both yield a measure of a general readiness to attack. However, since adult conspecifics may elicit long and often exhausting fights, whereas juveniles are simply chased and thus never cause any long-lasting aftereffects in the territorial male, the latter type of target appears to be a more suitable test stimulus to measure readiness to attack over longer periods of time. This is the reasoning behind the following experimental procedure.

An adult male is placed into an aquarium of 50 to 100 liters, and ten juveniles are provided to elicit occasional attacks. When no hiding places are available for the juveniles, they will uniformly distribute themselves about the whole aquarium and thus provide a randomized test stimulus for the adult male. Within a few days the adult male will have settled down in this environment, attacking the young fish at a moderate but regular rate.

To measure the effect of a given stimulus presentation on attack readiness the number of attacks against juveniles is recorded over the several minutes preceding and following the presentation. Since the juveniles are to serve as a constant test stimulus to measure attack readiness before and after stimulation, they should be prevented from seeing the stimulus presented to the adult male. (By severing their optic nerve, one can blind juveniles for the few weeks it takes this nerve to regenerate.)

Another territorial male, hidden behind an opaque partition, may be used to stimulate the resident male. This can be achieved by raising the opaque partition for several seconds while an additional glass partition prevents direct contact between the opponents. To further standardize this experiment a dummy resembling a conspecific opponent may be used instead. This dummy can be suspended above the aquarium and then lowered into the water to appear behind a glass partition. Figure 8.1 presents the experimental setup. Figure 8.2 shows the increase in attack rate caused by a 30-second presentation of a male dummy in the cichlid species *Pelmatochromis kribensis*.

The effect of a dummy presentation is characterized by two features. First, the initial increment in attack rate decays exponentially with a half-time of approximately two minutes (upper diagram in Figure 8.2).

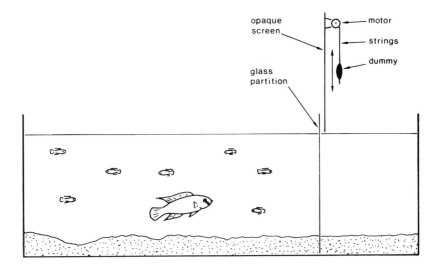

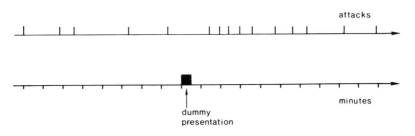

Figure 8.1 Experimental aquarium with a territorial male cichlid and several juveniles to the left of the glass partition. A dummy, hidden above the aquarium behind an opaque screen, can be lowered into the water by means of an electric motor to be presented to the male behind the glass partition. The lower part of the figure shows a recording of the male's attacks against juveniles. An increase in attack rate follows a 30-second presentation of the dummy.

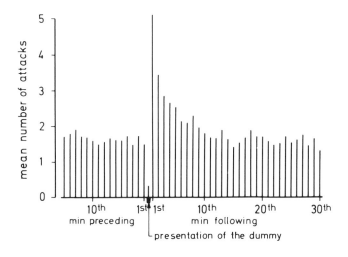

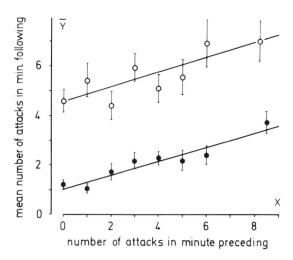

Figure 8.2 The rate of attacking in a male *Pelmatochromis kribensis* increases after a 30-second presentation of a dummy resembling a male conspecific. Upper diagram: Mean per-minute rate of attacking in 150 experiments. The increment in attack rate following the presentation of the dummy decays with a half-time of approximately two minutes. Lower diagram: Mean rate of attacking, $\bar{Y}$, in a subsequent one-minute period as a function of the rate X in the present one-minute period. Periods are separated by a 30-second interval. Presentation of the dummy during this interval leads to an additive increment in attack rate (open circles) over values obtained without stimulation (filled circles). Vertical bars indicate standard errors. Data with X values larger than six were rare; their mean X value is plotted on the abscissa. From Heiligenberg (1965).

Second, the mean attack rate counted after the dummy presentation is higher by a constant amount than what would be expected if no stimulus were presented (lower diagram). Moreover, when the present rate of attack is X, a mean rate $\bar{Y} = aX + c$ is to be expected in the subsequent period of time. Presentation of the stimulus between the present and subsequent period produces a mean rate $\bar{Y}_s = \bar{Y} + d = aX + c + d$, with d being the vertical distance between the parallel regression lines in the lower diagram of Figure 8.2. The effect of a given stimulus may thus be measured by the additive increment in attack rate d, which is independent of the prestimulatory level of attack rate.

Stimulus Patterns Affecting Attack Readiness

Cichlid fish show a variety of color patterns which may appear and disappear within minutes and are obviously correlated to certain behavioral states. For example, a given coloration A may indicate "fear," i.e., a high probability for fleeing and hiding, whereas another coloration B may characterize a highly aggressive territorial male. Such a male will switch from coloration B to coloration A when losing a fight against a stronger opponent. Figure 8.3 presents the patterns of coloration accompanying various behavioral states in the cichlid *Haplochromis burtoni*.

The fact that cichlid fish commonly change coloration during social encounters suggests that these color patterns serve a function in such interactions. Applying the experimental method outlined above, Leong presented different combinations of color patterns to adult territorial males of *Haplochromis burtoni*. The original thought of this investigation was to determine (1) which color patterns would affect the readiness to attack and (2) how combinations of such patterns would interact. Specifically, if the separately presented color patterns S_1 and S_2 change the attack rate by amounts d_1 and d_2, respectively, can the effect $d_{1,2}$ of the combined patterns $S_{1,2}$ be calculated from the amounts d_1 and d_2?

Experiments showed the following results. Only two color patterns have any significant effect on the attack rate. A black vertical eye-bar, part of the face pattern in territorial males (Figure 8.3), causes an increment in attack rate d_{bl} (Figure 8.4). A field of orange spots above the pectoral fin causes a decrement in attack rate $d_{or} < 0$ (Figure 8.5).

When both patterns are combined on a dummy, a total increment $d_{bl} + d_{or}$ is obtained (Figure 8.6). This value is still positive since the increment due to the black eye-bar exceeds the absolute value of the decrement due to the orange spots. Whereas the increment d_{bl} decays with a half-time of approximately three minutes, the decrement d_{or} decays with a half-time of approximately eleven minutes. This demonstrates that the time course of the aftereffects caused by such stimuli depends on the type of stimulus presented and therefore cannot be attributed to features of the final common motor output. Certain stimulus patterns thus elicit excitatory or inhibitory processes that are characterized by particular amplitudes and time constants of decay. Such processes may be additively superimposed if the corresponding stimulus patterns are presented simultaneously.

When a male *Haplochromis* is isolated for several weeks together with

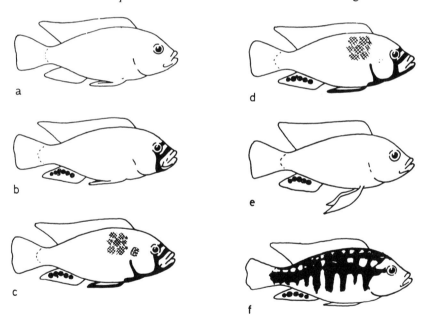

Figure 8.3 Color patterns in *Haplochromis burtoni*. Juveniles and females are uniformly grey (a). A young male ready to establish territory shows a black head pattern and yellowish spots on his anal fin (b). A territorial male develops additional black coloration on his chin and pelvic fins and a field of orange spots above his pectoral fins(c). A black opercular spot disappears during spawning (d). A frightened male turns immediately pale (e) and develops a black-cross pattern when taking cover (f). From Leong (1969).

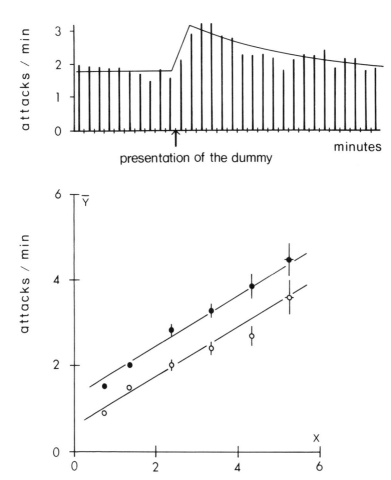

Figure 8.4 The rate of attacking in a male *Haplochromis burtoni* increases after 30-second presentation of a fish dummy with a vertical black eye-bar. Upper diagram: Mean per-minute rate of attacking in approximately 150 experiments with several specimens. The increment in attack rate following the presentation of the dummy decays with a half-time of approximately three minutes. Lower diagram: Mean rate of attacking, $\bar{Y}$, in subsequent five-minute period as a function of rate X in the present five-minute period. Present and subsequent five-minute periods are separated by a 30-second interval. Presentation of the dummy during this interval leads to an additive increment in attack rate (filled circles) as compared to values obtained without stimulation (open circles). Data are grouped according to different ranges of their X values. Mean X and Y values and standard errors are plotted. Data from Heiligenberg et al. (1972).

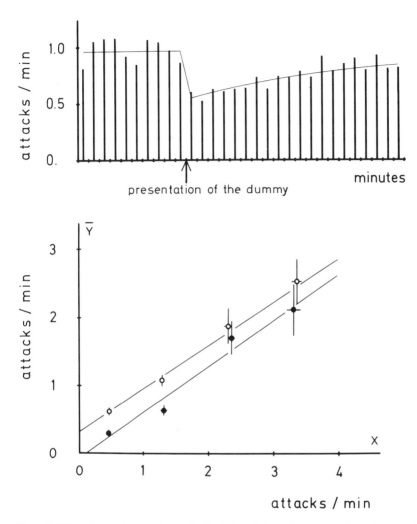

Figure 8.5 The rate of attacking in a male *Haplochromis burtoni* decreases after a 30-second presentation of a fish dummy with orange spots above the pectoral fins. Presentation as in Figure 8.4 with approximately 120 experiments on several specimens. The decrement in attack rate decays with a half-time of approximately 11 minutes. Unpublished data by Heiligenberg and Kramer.

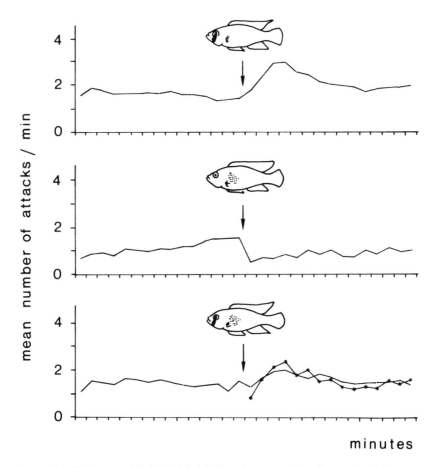

Figure 8.6 The incremental effect of the black eye-bar pattern (top diagram) and the decremental effect of the orange-spots pattern (center) are additively superimposed when both patterns are presented on the same dummy (bottom). The curve expected under the assumption of additive superposition is marked by asterisks and hardly differs from the true data in the bottom diagram. Average per-minute rates of attacking were calculated from original data of Leong (1969). Since dummies were presented repeatedly at half-hour periods, the animals recovered insufficiently from the slow inhibitory process between successive presentations. This explains the small rise in attack rate during the prestimulatory period in the center diagram. Dummies were presented at longer periods in the more recent data in Figure 8.5. The number of experiments underlying the top, center, and bottom diagrams are approximately 150, 80, and 150, respectively.

a number of small test fish, its attack rate will decline and eventually approach zero unless the animal is allowed to encounter conspecifics or at least dummies resembling territorial males. It appears that regular stimulation is required to maintain a sufficiently high level of attack readiness. This was demonstrated in the following experiment.

In the experimental setup described above a male cichlid was isolated with ten juveniles for at least six weeks, so that its mean attack rate almost reached zero. Then, on ten successive days, a dummy with a vertical black eye-bar was presented every 15 minutes for 30 seconds, from 9 A.M. to 5 P.M. After these ten days all stimulus presentation ceased. As is demonstrated in Figure 8.7, the attack rate rose during the ten days of stimulation and then slowly returned to its prestimulatory near-zero level. No such effect was encountered when a dummy without

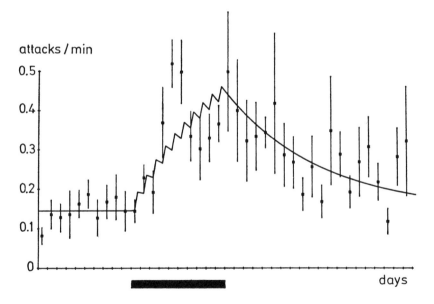

Figure 8.7 A long-term increment in attack rate caused by repeated presentations of the vertical black eye-bar pattern. After single males of *Haplochromis burtoni* had not been exposed to conspecifics or dummies for several weeks, their rate of attacks against small juveniles reached a very low level. Presentations of dummies at 15-minute intervals over a period of ten successive days (bar underlining abscissa) led to a gradual rise in attack rate. This increment decayed again with a half-time of seven days. The graph shows average data of four specimens observed for a few hours every day. The continuous line represents a long-term model process. From Heiligenberg and Kramer (1972).

a vertical black eye-bar was presented instead. This demonstrates that specific rather than general stimuli are required to maintain a high level of attack readiness in isolated cichlid males.

To explain the slow rise and decay in attack rate shown in Figure 8.7 in an elementary manner one could postulate that each dummy presentation causes a small additive increment A in the attack rate which decays with a long half-time T. When successive stimuli are presented, the elicited increments are superimposed on one another and gradually lead to a build-up in the attack rate. According to this model increments would be added each day between 9 A.M. and 5 P.M., followed by a slow decay during the night. This would lead to a stepwise build-up in attack rate over the ten consecutive days of stimulation and a subsequent slow return to the baseline level with a half-time T. The continuous line in the diagram of Figure 8.7 represents this model process in which the increment A in attack rate caused by a single dummy presentation and the half-time T of the subsequent decay process were optimized to fit the data. The values for A and T are 0.0015 attacks/min and seven days, respectively.

An Analogue Model of Short- and Long-Term Processes Affecting the Readiness to Attack

So far three processes have been described that affect the readiness to attack. The vertical black eye-bar causes a short-term incremental process that decays with a half-time of approximately three minutes and a long-term incremental process that decays with a half-time of seven days. The amplitude of this long-term process, however, is so small that it can only be detected after consecutive stimulation has led to a gradual build-up in attack rate. Finally the field of orange spots above the pectoral fins causes a decremental short-term process that decays with a half-time of approximately eleven minutes. These processes, once elicited by their corresponding stimulus patterns, are superimposed upon the present level of attack readiness R (Figure 8.8).

There seem to be additional processes of this kind contributing to the total "amount" of attack readiness that are elicited by chemical or mechanical stimuli rather than by visual signals. Also, an internal variable I of unknown origin is considered to cause fluctuations in attack

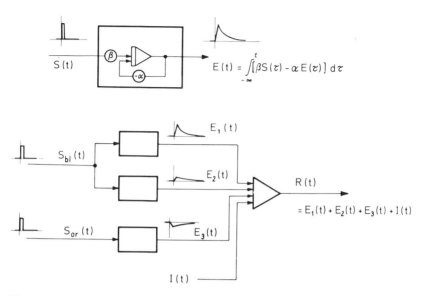

Figure 8.8. Analogue model representing the effect of certain stimulus patterns on the readiness to attack. The upper diagram shows a circuit generating a process E which decays with a rate constant α after a short stimulus presentation S. The lower diagram shows short- and long-term excitatory processes, E_1 and E_2, elicited by the black eye-bar pattern and an inhibitory process, E_3, elicited by orange spots above pectorals. I represents an internal variable contributing to the attack readiness R. From Heiligenberg (1974a).

rate that are independent of external stimulation. However, since the readiness to attack sinks to a very low level in the absence of such stimuli, this internal component I does not play a major role. (A detailed presentation of this system is given in Heiligenberg, 1974a.) A stochastic analysis of spontaneous fluctuations in the rate of attacking and other behaviors revealed that the internal component I in Figure 8.8 can be represented as a combination of at least four orthogonal random processes that control different behaviors to different extents (Heiligenberg, 1974b).

The phenomena described in this paper may be viewed from a different aspect and may be explained in different terms. One could argue that a territorial male cichlid will *habituate* to the continuous presence of small test fish and thus attack at a low rate. The presentation of certain stimuli would *dishabituate* the animal and thus lead to a temporary increase in attack rate. Dishabituation or "sensitization" is considered to be a process independent of the process of habituation (Groves and Thompson, 1970), a notion supported by recent studies on *Aplysia* neurons (Carew and Kandel, 1974). The two excitatory processes E_1 and E_2 in Figure 8.8 may be viewed as sensitization processes of this kind.

The Biological Significance of External Control of Readiness to Attack
Little is known about the behavior of *Haplochromis burtoni* in its natural habitat. Therefore all statements about the significance of different color patterns with respect to aggression are based on aquarium observations (Leong, 1969). Immature animals live in schools and are uniformly grey. Young males reaching maturity frequently show a black vertical eye-bar and eventually separate from their school to settle down in a territory. Adult males live in neighboring territories and commonly fight each other on their boundaries. A colony of such territories may occupy the whole bottom area of the aquarium. A young male trying to establish an additional territory will, because of its black head pattern, raise the aggressiveness in the resident males and thus draw attacks. This in turn may lead to its expulsion and thus prevent overcrowding of the colony. However, when a young male succeeds in settling down in a new territory, it will develop orange spots above its pectoral fins within days. These spots characterize resident territorial males. Their negative effect on readiness to attack should buffer the excitatory effect of the black eye-bar pattern and thus maintain aggressiveness among residents at a moderate level.

    Haplochromis burtoni mainly attacks conspecific males, whereas females and juveniles are tolerated to some extent. Attacking behavior serves to secure a territory into which females are led for spawning. Only a territory of sufficient size will prevent interference by other males. There is thus little "need" for a *Haplochromis* male to be aggressive in the absence of male competitors. The main function of the black eye-bar pattern appears to be to raise the readiness to attack whenever it is needed.

Summary
The behavioral experiments described in this paper have demonstrated the influence of certain visual stimulus patterns on the state of aggression

in fish. Excitatory and inhibitory processes were investigated that can easily be linked to similar, known neuronal processes in other systems. The quantitative method applied in this study could be used to analyze various other aspects of aggression, such as the effect of early experience, the significance of the social environment, the role of hormones, etc. Such studies should eventually yield a complete picture of the aggressive system in this fish and might suggest basic principles that hold for higher animals as well.

References
Carew, T. J., and Kandel, E. R. 1974. Synaptic analysis of the interrelationships between behavioral modifications in *Aplysia*. In M. V. L. Bennett, ed., *Synaptic Transmission and Neuronal Interaction*. New York: Raven Press.

Courchesne, E., and Barlow, G. W. 1971. Effect of isolation on components of aggressive and other behavior in the Hermit Crab, *Pagurus samuelis*. *Z. Vergl. Physiol.* 75:32–48.

Eibl-Eibesfeldt, I. 1970. *Ethology, the biology of behavior*. New York: Holt, Rinehart and Winston.

Franck, D., and Wilhelmi, U. 1973. Veränderungen der aggressiven Handlungsbereitschaft männlicher Schwertträger, *Xiphophorus helleri,* nach sozialer Isolation. *Experientia* 29:896.

Groves, Ph. M., and Thompson, R. F. 1970. Habituation: A dual-process theory. *Psychol. Rev.* 77:419–450.

Heiligenberg, W. 1965. The effect of external stimuli on the attack readiness of a cichlid fish. *Z. Vergl. Physiol.* 49:459–464.

Heiligenberg, W. 1973. Random processes describing the occurrence of behavioral patterns in a cichlid fish. *Anim. Behav.* 21:169–182.

Heiligenberg, W. 1974a. Processes governing behavioral states of readiness. In *Advances in the study of behavior*, vol. 5. New York: Academic Press.

Heiligenberg, W. 1974b. A stochastic analysis of fish behavior. In D. McFarland, ed., *Motivational control systems analysis*. New York: Academic Press.

Heiligenberg, W., and Kramer, U. 1972. Aggressiveness as a function of external stimulation. *J. Comp. Physiol.* 77:332–340.

Heiligenberg, W., Kramer, U., and Schulz, V. 1972. The angular orientation of the black eye-bar in *Haplochromis burtoni* and its relevance to aggressivity. *Z. Vergl. Physiol.* 76:168–176.

Hinde, R. A. 1969. The bases of aggression in animals. *J. Psychosom. Res.* 13:213–219.

Leong, C. Y. 1969. The quantitative effect of releasers on the attack readiness of the fish, *Haplochromis burtoni. Z. Vergl. Physiol.* 65:29–50.

Lorenz, K. Z. 1963. *Das sogenannte Böse.* Vienna: Borotha Verlag.

Rasa, O. A. E. 1970. A demonstration of appetitive behavior for aggression in the coral fish, *Microspathodon chrysurus.* Dissertation, University of Oxford.

Scott, J. P. 1968. In A. Montague, ed., *Man and aggression.* New York: Oxford Univ. Press.

Scott, J. P. 1971. Theoretical issues concerning the origin and causes of fighting. In B. E. Eleftherious and J. P. Scott, eds., *The physiology of aggression and defeat.* New York: Plenum Press.

9

A Model System for Neurophysiological Investigations of Behavioral Plasticity

Dennis L. Glanzman, Timothy J. Teyler, and Richard F. Thompson

An analysis of the neural correlates of the behavior of organisms is complicated by the fact that organisms displaying behaviors of interest to psychobiologists are also the most biologically complex. This level of complexity is a severe limitation to the investigation of the mechanisms underlying the behavior. It thus seems advantageous to limit the domain of study; the limitations can be imposed both upon the degree of behavioral complexity required of the organism and on the biological complexity of the preparation. The former limitation is effected by the utilization of simpler paradigms such as habituation and classical conditioning, and the latter by employing simple biological preparations such as spinal cord or invertebrate ganglia.

To analyze completely a particular behavior it often becomes necessary either to restrict the nature of the response or, more commonly, to limit the stimuli presented to and received by the experimental animal. These two restrictions are often closely interrelated. Thus the approach employed may be considered to be a "model paradigm" of a behavior or process occurring in a more complex natural environment. Similarly, by reducing the biological complexity of the experimental subject, one can obtain detailed information of a more fundamental nature. The excitatory and inhibitory influences upon a given cell, for example, are more easily studied in such reduced systems. Information of this type may then be generalized to the intact animal, and postulates made as to the possible physiological mechanisms underlying more biologically complex behaviors or functions. The two approaches may be used either independently or in conjunction.

Experimental psychology has long employed classical and

D. L. Glanzman, T. J. Teyler, and R. F. Thompson, Laboratory of Psychobiology, Department of Psychology and Social Relations, Harvard University, Cambridge, MA, 02138.

instrumental conditioning as laboratory analogues of natural learning. In classical conditioning an initially meaningless or nonrelevant stimulus is presented to the subject, closely followed in time by a stimulus that initially elicits a response. After repeated presentations, or pairings, of these stimuli the initially meaningless (conditioned) stimulus, CS, elicits a response previously occurring only to the second (unconditioned) stimulus, US. The resulting response to the CS is termed a conditioned response, CR, and is the paradigm employed in many animal learning studies. A second type of "model paradigm" is instrumental conditioning. In one example of instrumental conditioning the subject is given an initially meaningless stimulus, such as a light flash or a tone burst, followed closely in time by an aversive stimulus, such as an electric shock. In the intervening period the subject is allowed to perform some task, such as walking through a doorway to the "safe" side of the testing chamber, which results in avoidance of the aversive stimulus. Such instrumental avoidance paradigms are also often used as model paradigms of behavioral situations. Similarly, and perhaps even more to the point, instrumental reward learning in animals is both rapid and "natural," and may be formalized in relatively simple terms by application of the Law of Effect (Herrnstein, 1970).

Although there is an objection raised by some investigators that model paradigms are somewhat "artificial," they do provide examples of learned behavior that are more easily quantified than are some "natural" functions. Moreover, habituation, which is a decrement in response to repeated presentations of unchanging stimuli, is very frequently found in "natural" settings. Additional power is available to the study of the neurology of learning by application of the model-systems approach to both behavior and biology simultaneously. Such is the subject of this paper: model preparations and model paradigms in the study of behavioral plasticity or learning.

Model Preparations
The model preparations that have been used for the study of learning can be classified into three mutually nonexclusive types of biological preparation: model systems, simple systems, and reduced systems. We will provide arbitrary definitions to illustrate distinctions.

A *model* system is one in which there exists implied physiological and behavioral relationships to the referent. For example, the flexion of an individual muscle or muscle group in a restrained intact animal may be an ideal choice as a model system, since the physiological condition of the animal is unchanged and a specific muscle contraction being measured occurs equally well in restrained and freely moving animals. The advantages of such a preparation are manifold: one is not subject to the restrictions and limitations imposed by anesthesia, paralysis, or surgical alteration. This type of model system provides perhaps the most nearly "normal" analogue to the natural physiological activity of the intact animal. A model system also allows analysis of physiological events occurring within a chronic preparation. However, it is often poorly suited for the examination of the more molecular phenomena, such as biochemical alterations occurring during learning.

Simple systems most commonly involve the invertebrate nervous system, where the total neuron population may number in the hundreds rather than in the billions. Preparations often used by neurophysiologists and behaviorists involve the leech, lobster, crayfish, *Aplysia*, squid, earthworm, and cockroach. Each of these animals has a very limited nervous system or nerve net, several orders of magnitude smaller in number (and therefore presumably in complexity) than the vertebrate nervous system. Although this system offers many advantages in terms of biological simplicity, it may not be a good behavioral model of learning occurring in higher animals since invertebrates may be incapable of the more complex forms of learning. They are, however, eminently useful in the examination of simple learning-like tasks, such as habituation to tactile stimulation (Pinsker et al., 1970), and possibly even of discrimination learning, and in the electrophysiological and biochemical analysis of behavioral changes.

A *reduced* preparation is one in which either a specific piece of tissue has been removed and kept in vitro for further examination or most afferents (and possibly efferents) have been severed in situ in order to render a less complex preparation in terms of inputs and outputs. This technique is often combined with one or both of the preceding systems. In the isolated ganglia of *Aplysia* (Castellucci et al., 1970; Kandel and

Gardner, 1972) one finds reduced, simple systems wherein lie a relatively small number of individual neurons, which exhibit electrophysiological correlates of behavioral phenomena observed in the intact animal. The isolated spinal cord of the frog offers a reduced model of the vertebrate central nervous system in which a detailed examination of the correlates of habituation has been made across a monosynaptic pathway (Farel et al., 1973). In the reduced system it is imperative to demonstrate that the phenomena under investigation have strong correlations with the behavior of the intact animal, as in the case of the reflex arc in the cat spinal cord (Prosser and Hunter, 1936; Thompson and Spencer, 1966; Eccles, 1964) and the gill-withdrawal reflex of *Aplysia* (Kupfermann et al., 1970; Castellucci et al., 1970).

A good model preparation (including model, simple, and reduced systems) must possess many of the features of the intact animal if it is to yield useful information about the mechanisms of learning. For example, in electrophysiological investigations it must be demonstrated that the responses of the isolated or altered tissue represent faithfully the responses of comparable structures in the intact animal. Discrepancies in the responses of isolated vs. intact tissue must be accounted for in terms of both anatomical and physiological changes (for example, isolation of a slab of neural tissue from the rest of the animal may result in the removal of normally inhibitory influences, yielding a system more excitable and more highly responsive than that examined in vivo). Similarly, in biochemical situations the ability of the tissue to carry out normal metabolic and catabolic functions must be demonstrated for the duration of the experiment.

Model Paradigms

A model paradigm should possess the same advantages as do the model preparations.

1. The procedure should be *simple* so that a limited potential for response complexity is inherent in the design. Procedural simplicity is crucial when used in conjunction with a model preparation which itself may be incapable of responding appropriately in complex paradigms.

2. The paradigm must be *robust*. Interanimal differences should be as limited as possible.

3. For physiological examinations it is often essential that the behavioral change be produced *rapidly* (during the course of recording from a single cell, for example).

4. The paradigm must be amenable to the application of *control* procedures to rule out extraneous behavioral changes.

5. On occasion the pairing of a CS and a US will result in a response to the CS that is not attributable to the pairing of the two stimuli. In these cases any CS-like stimulus introduced at any time will evoke a response. By definition these "pseudoconditional" responses are not the result of a temporal pairing of CS and US but represent nonassociative alterations in behavior. In this case the incorporation of an explicitly unpaired CS and US group and a group receiving random CS and US presentations will satisfy the control requirements for most classical conditioning experiments (Rescorla, 1967).

6. Finally, for maximum utility it is desirable that the paradigm be applicable over a wide *ontogenetic and phylogenetic range*.

The model paradigms that have been employed in neurobehavioral studies of plasticity can be divided into two categories: associative and nonassociative. Of the two the nonassociative paradigm is the simpler. We here refer to *habituation* or *sensitization* paradigms wherein single stimuli are presented repeatedly. In habituation the responses of the organism, both behavioral and physiological, decrease as a function of repeated stimulations; in sensitization they increase. A critical feature to note is that a new response is not established; rather an existing response is modified. Thus habituation or sensitization paradigms are simpler in form and effect than associative paradigms.

Associative paradigms are generally of two varieties: classical conditioning and instrumental conditioning. Both feature the temporal association of two unrelated events. In classical conditioning an initially neutral stimulus is repeatedly paired in time with a meaningful stimulus in such a way that a response develops to the first stimulus. In instrumental conditioning the organism receives reinforcing stimulation (either positive or negative) contingent upon its production of some behavior. The behavior will be modified as a function of the nature of the associated stimulation. In both cases a preparation is required that will show changes specific to two events *related in time.* Conditioning parameters thus assume a level of complexity higher than those of nonassociative paradigms. As examples of the use of these model paradigms one could cite classical conditioning occurring within a spinal-reflex arc (Patterson, Cegavske, and Thompson, 1973) and classical conditioning of the nictitating-membrane response in rabbit (Coleman and Gormezano, 1971).

Models for the Study of Habituation

Two model preparations used in this laboratory are the acute spinal cat and the isolated spinal cord of frog (both are reduced model systems). The model paradigm is that of habituation/sensitization. These model approaches are particularly applicable to studies of the neuronal bases of plasticity since they permit the testing of specific hypotheses regarding the neural mechanisms underlying changes in neuronal activity.

Several years ago Thompson and Spencer (1966) characterized nine parametric features of habituation common to many preparations, mostly occurring within the vertebrate central nervous system. Seven of these characteristics deal with response habituation (time course and recovery, effect of repeated series, effect of stimulus intensity and frequency, stimulus generalization, and below-zero habituation). Two of the features deal with response sensitization (dishabituation and habituation of dishabituation). Examination of these parameters in specific instances, such as habituation of the hindlimb flexion reflex in acute spinal cat (Groves et al., 1969a,b, 1970; Glanzman et al., 1972), have illustrated the value of this preparation in examining the simplest form of learning. This model consists, quite simply, of an anesthetized cat with a spinal transection, at the level of the twelfth thoracic vertebra, that removes all ascending and, more importantly, all descending influences from the brain. A dorsal spinal laminectomy is performed over vertebral segments L5 to S1, allowing penetration of both stimulating and recording microelectrodes into spinal grey while maintaining the spinal blood supply. The superficial and deep peroneal nerves are used for stimulating and recording. The caudal tendon of the tibialis anterior muscle is tied to a strain gauge to monitor muscle contraction. Finally surgical needles are inserted into the foot pads to be used as stimulating electrodes. The animal is rigidly fixed into a spinal stereotaxic apparatus, and experimentation is commenced.

A behavioral situation is closely duplicated when the foot pad is stimulated electrically and the resulting muscle flexion amplitude is recorded. Monitoring afferent and efferent volleys from the peroneal nerves has demonstrated that the response decrement obtained during habituation occurs central to both receptors and effectors. Stimulation of the superficial peroneal nerve at intensities that lead to afferent volleys in the dorsal root of a similar amplitude to those of direct sensory stimulation (foot shock) produces a habituating response in the ventral root that parallels foot-pad stimulation responses.

Groves and coworkers (1970) tested the excitability of cutaneous afferent terminals during habituation and sensitization in an attempt to evaluate presynaptic inhibition as a mechanism of habituation. Using Wall's (1958) technique of stimulating afferent terminals and recording antidromic responses in the dorsal root, they demonstrated that there was no increase in antidromic volley during habituation and no decrease during sensitization. This study thus demonstrated that presynaptic inhibition of afferent fibers does not underlie habituation.

Spencer and coworkers (1966) found no change in the resting-membrane potential or excitability of motoneurons during habituation, but they did report an occasional background depolarization following a strong dishabituating stimulus. The apparent lack of hyperpolarization during habituation training argues against postsynaptic inhibition as a mediator of habituation. Furthermore intravenously administered picrotoxin or strychnine, which depress many forms of pre- and postsynaptic inhibition (Eccles, 1964), did not alter the occurrence of habituation when stimulus intensities were reduced to yield preinjection control responses (Thompson and Spencer, 1966).

A rather broad localization of habituation had thus been made in the spinal-reflex arc, occurring somewhere between afferent terminals and motoneurons, and two possible mechanisms of habituation had been eliminated. Since neither pre- nor postsynaptic inhibition appear to be a necessary and sufficient condition for habituation to occur, Spencer and coworkers (1966) and Thompson and Spencer (1966) proposed that some form of polysynaptic-homosynaptic depression operates within the interneuronal pathway mediating flexor twitch.

In subsequent studies discharge patterns of interneurons in the spinal grey were studied during the course of simultaneous sensitization and habituation training of the hindlimb flexor response in acute spinal cat. In brief two categories of interneurons were found that exhibited plasticity of response to repeated stimulation. One category—type H—exhibits only decrement, regardless of whether or not the reflex response shows sensitization. An example is given in Figure 9.1. These interneurons are found in Rexed (1954) layers I–V and always have short latency responses. The other category of "plastic" interneurons—type S—shows an incremental response followed by decrement and tends to parallel the course of the reflex quite closely. These interneurons typically are found more ventrally, in layers V–VII, and have longer onset latencies than type-H interneurons.

These two categories of interneurons were taken as prototypical of underlying central processes of sensitization and habituation, and a "dual-process" theory of habituation was thus developed (Groves and Thompson, 1970, 1973; Thompson et al., 1973). This theory, based on a simplified model approach, permitted successful postdiction and prediction of a wide variety of behavioral and neuronal phenomena of habituation. However, it "failed" in the sense that the critical synapses where plasticity of response to repeated stimulation developed could not be identified with certainty and, hence, could not be analyzed in terms of mechanisms.

Consequently a still simpler model system of habituation in the vertebrate central nervous system was developed in this laboratory—the isolated spinal cord of the frog (Farel et al., 1973). This preparation offers one major advantage over the acute spinal cat: there exists a known monosynaptic pathway from the lateral column to the motoneurons of the lumbosacral cord in frog that exhibits the characteristics of habituation of Thompson and Spencer (1966).

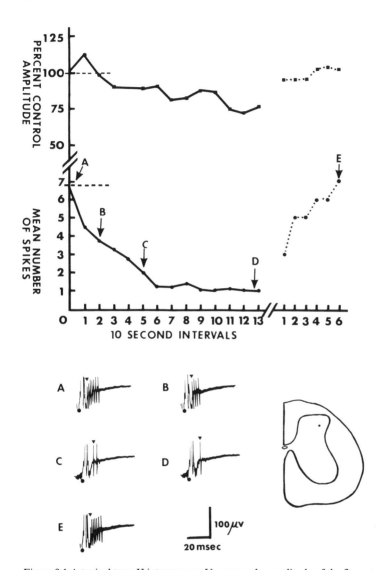

Figure 9.1 A typical type-H interneuron. Upper graph: amplitude of the flexor twitch of the tibialis anterior muscle showing sensitization followed by habituation and spontaneous recovery. Lower graph: mean number of spikes per stimulus of a simultaneously recorded interneuron. Note that the interneuron shows only a progressive decrease in evoked discharges even during behavioral sensitization. The position of the electrode tip is shown at lower right. Sample oscilloscope tracings are shown in A–E. From Groves and Thompson (1973).

In this preparation the entire spinal cord caudal to the cerebellum is dissected from the unanesthetized (pithed or decapitated) frog and is kept electrophysiologically functional for periods of up to 24 hours. The spinal cord is mounted on its side in a recording chamber and is constantly superfused with fortified, oxygenated frog Ringer's solution. Ventral roots nine and ten are draped over platinum stimulating/recording electrodes and are coated with mineral oil to prevent drying. A bipolar stimulating electrode is laid against the descending lateral-column (LC) fiber tract, and a pial dissection is made over the motoneuron pool. Glass micropipettes are lowered stereo-taxically into the motoneuron pool until a cell is encountered and penetrated, identified as a motoneuron (MN) by antidromic stimulation of the ventral root (VR), and tested for responsiveness to LC stimulation. Responses are then measured to LC stimulation at rates of 0.1 to 0.5 per second, and the resulting action potential or excitatory postsynaptic potential (EPSP) is recorded photographically from the oscilloscope face. Data are also recorded on magnetic tape for subsequent computer analysis. The observed decrease in response of motoneurons (EPSP) to LC stimulation is open to several lines of interpretation. Decrements of this sort occurring in other preparations have been termed habituation, depression, antifacilitation, fatigue, and, in long-term observations, degeneration.

An example of habituation of the monosynaptic VR response to repeated LC stimulation is shown in Figure 9.2. A single weak electrical pulse is given to the lateral column every five seconds. Pronounced habituation develops within five to ten trials. Recovery from such training can last as long as fifteen to twenty minutes after only fifty trials—a prolonged decrement for a monosynaptic response.

Figure 9.3 schematically represents four possible heterosynaptic neural circuits which may underlie the response decrement. Recurrent collaterals from motoneuron axons may activate interneurons, which could in turn affect polarizations of pre- or postsynaptic elements. Alternatively, afferent collaterals may cause interneuronal inhibition of the same structures. Circuits involving recurrent collaterals from moto-neurons (9.3A, 9.3B) may be eliminated as habituation mechanisms by one test—repeated activation of motoneurons by antidromic VR stimu-lation. If these circuits were mediating habituation, one would find

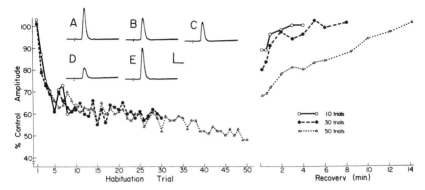

Figure 9.2 Habituation and recovery of ventral-root response to 10, 30, and 50 lateral-column stimuli presented at 0.2-sec intervals. The graph represents means drawn from three preparations, each of which was run in each stimulus condition. Note the exponential decline in response amplitude and the inverse relation between number of stimulus presentations and recovery rate. Inset: example of the decrement of ventral-root response to repeated lateral-column stimulation. Responses are shown to the 1st (A), 2nd (B), 3rd (C), and 10th (D) stimuli of a train of 10 stimuli presented to lateral column. Recovery two minutes later (E) is also shown. From Farel et al. (1973).

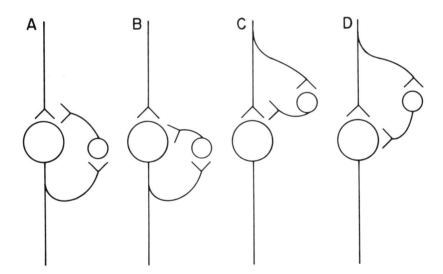

Figure 9.3 Possible heterosynaptic mechanisms of habituation involving interneurons. Recurrent collaterals from motoneuron axons could excite interneurons, which in turn exert presynaptic influences (A), presumably through depolarization of axon terminals or hyperpolarization of the motoneuron membrane. Afferent collaterals could also involve interneurons to exert either presynaptic actions (C) or postsynaptic actions (D). From Farel et al. (1973).

a response decrement with repeated stimulation since the antidromic action potential would invade the axon collateral and activate the inhibitory pathway. In no instance was this observed in the isolated spinal cord of the frog, even at frequencies and intensities of stimulation that produced marked habituation when delivered by orthodromic LC pathways (Farel et al., 1973). Results of this type of experiment are illustrated in Figure 9.4.

The two remaining possibilities were also tested, as in the case of the spinal cat. In accordance with Wall's (1958) technique a large (25-μ) stimulating electrode was lowered into the motoneuron pool and conditioning stimuli were given in advance of regular LC stimulating pulses. Antidromic responses of LC fibers were recorded after microelectrode stimulation of the motoneuron pool, and orthodromic VR responses to LC stimulation were used as a measure of the habituation of the motoneurons (Figure 9.5). This test allowed relative measurements to be made of LC-terminal excitability. If presynaptic inhibition (Figures 9.3A and 9.3C) were a mechanism of habituation, one would expect an *increase* in the amplitude of the antidromically elicited response in LC fibers due to a depolarization of LC terminals leading to a relative decrease in their response threshold. At no time was this observed in our investigations.

A final test of postsynaptic inhibition was made in the following way.

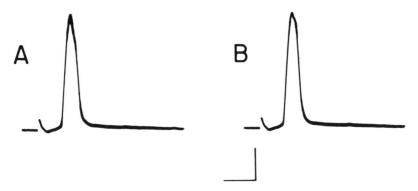

Figure 9.4 Ventral-root responses to lateral-column stimulation evoked before (A) and after (B) twenty stimuli delivered antidromically to the ventral root at 0.5-sec intervals. Calibration: 2 mv, 4 msec. From Farel et al. (1973).

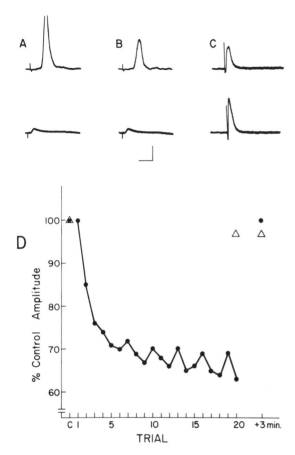

Figure 9.5 Test for changes in excitability of LC terminals. A, top: VR response to first LC stimulus of a train of twenty stimuli delivered at 0.2-msec intervals. Bottom: response recorded from dissected LC fibers to a stimulus applied through a glass-coated tungsten microelectrode in the motoneuron pool. Stimulus presented 1 sec after that eliciting the VR response shown above. B, top: VR response to 20th LC stimulus. Bottom: response to pulse applied through the microelectrode 1 sec after that eliciting the VR response shown above. Note that, although the VR response to LC stimulation has declined, the antidromic response to activation of LC terminals is unchanged. C, top: response recorded on DR to a stimulus applied through microelectrode in superficial regions of dorsal horn. Bottom: as above, but evoked 20 msec after an orthodromic stimulus had been applied to that DR. Note that the response elicited by terminal activation is potentiated, indicating increased terminal excitability. D: data are mean values from ten preparations in which terminal excitability was examined. Black circles indicate VR responses to LC stimulations and triangles indicate antidromic responses of LC fibers elicited by microelectrodes in the motoneuron pool. Calibration: A and B, top: 2 mv, 4 msec; A and B, bottom: 0.2 mv, 4 msec; C: 0.2 mv, 4 msec.

Motoneuron responses to dorsal-root (DR) stimulation were recorded before and after habituation of the LC-MN pathway. Brookhart and coworkers (1959) have described the interactions between DR and LC volleys on the VR response, and Fadiga and Brookhart (1960) have demonstrated that these two systems converge upon the same motoneurons. If postsynaptic inhibition (Figures 9.3B and 9.3D) were a mechanism of habituation, one would expect a generalization of response decrement to DR inputs from LC habituation since the postsynaptic cell (MN) would, presumably, maintain the reduced capacity for response through hyperpolarization. As Figure 9.6 demonstrates, there was no consistent decrement in motoneuron response to DR stimulation following severe habituation of the LC-MN response.

The habituation observed in this monosynaptic system "appears to be the result of some processes of homosynaptic depression limited to the synapses of the lateral-column fibers on motoneuron somata and

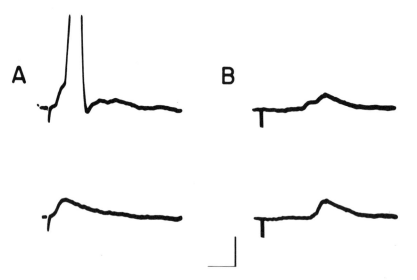

Figure 9.6 Intracellularly recorded responses of a motoneuron to LC and DR stimulation before and after habituation to repeated LC stimulation. A, top: control response of motoneuron to LC stimulation. B, top: control response of motoneuron to DR stimulation applied 5 sec after response in A. A, bottom: last response of motoneuron to a series of 20 stimuli delivered to LC at 0.5-sec intervals. B, bottom: response to DR stimulus applied 5 sec after last LC stimulus. Calibration: 4 mv, 10 msec. From Farel et al. (1973).

proximal dendrites activated by the lateral-column stimulus" (Farel et al., 1973). The further localization of a form of habituation to a single histologically identifiable type of synapse provides an excellent model system in a reduced preparation for the more molecular investigations of the mechanisms of habituation in the vertebrate central nervous system.

Similar decrements have been reported at single synapses in certain invertebrate preparations: in the abdominal ganglion of *Aplysia* (Castellucci et al., 1970; Kupfermann et al., 1970; Pinsker et al., 1970; see also Kandel and Spencer, 1968) and at an afferent synapse on an interneuron in crayfish (Zucker, 1972). In these instances the mechanism appears to be a form of homosynaptic depression, as is true for our vertebrate monosynaptic model system. Indeed the many, varied preparations in which habituation has been studied all provide results consistent with the notion that habituation is a phenomenon of synaptic depression intrinsic to the synapses being activated. The fact that habituation has shown the same type of mechanism whenever it has been studied at a single synapse, and the equally important fact that the phenomena of habituation exhibit a most impressive degree of similarity across several phyla from at least *Aplysia* to man, support the hypothesis of a common neuronal mechanism of synaptic depression. Indeed it may be fairly stated that we have a much clearer understanding of the fundamental mechanism underlying habituation than we do for any other form of behavioral plasticity or learning, thanks in large measure to the successful application of the "model approach."

References

Brookhart, J. M., Machne, X., and Fadiga, E. 1959. Patterns of motor neuron discharge in the frog. *Arch. Ital. Biol.* 97:53–67.

Castellucci, V., Pinsker, H., Kupfermann, I., and Kandel, E. 1970. Neural mechanisms of habituation and dishabituation of the gill-withdrawal reflex in *Aplysia. Science* 167:1745–1748.

Coleman, S. R., and Gormezano, I. 1971. Classical conditioning of the rabbit's (oryctolagus cuniculus) nictitating membrane response under symmetrical CS-US interval shifts. *J. Comp. Physiol. Psychol.*, 77:447–455.

Eccles, J. C. 1965. *The physiology of synapses.* New York: Springer-Verlag.

Fadiga, E., and Brookhart, J. M. 1960. Monosynaptic activation of different portions of the motor neuron membrane. *Am. J. Physiol.* 198:693–703.

Farel, P. B., Glanzman, D. L., and Thompson, R. F. 1973. Habituation of a monosynaptic response in the vertebrate central nervous system: lateral column-motoneuron pathway in isolated frog spinal cord. *J. Neurophysiol.* 36:1117–1130.

Glanzman, D. L., Groves, P. M., and Thompson, R. F. 1972. Stimulus generalization of habituation in spinal interneurons. *Physiol. Behav.* 8:155–158.

Groves, P. M., DeMarco, R., and Thompson, R. F. 1969a. Habituation and sensitization of spinal interneuron activity in acute spinal cat. *Brain Res.* 14:521–525.

Groves, P. M., Glanzman, D. L., Patterson, M. M., and Thompson, R. F. 1970. Excitability of cutaneous afferent terminals during habituation and sensitization in acute spinal cat. *Brain Res.* 18:388–392.

Groves, P. M., Lee, D., and Thompson, R. F. 1969b. Effects of stimulus frequency and intensity on habituation and sensitization in acute spinal cat. *Physiol. Behav.* 4:383–388.

Groves, P. M., and Thompson, R. F. 1973. A dual-process theory of habituation: neural mechanisms. In H. V. S. Peeke and M. J. Herz, eds., *Habituation.* New York: Academic Press.

Harris, J. D. 1943. Habituatory response decrement in the intact organism. *Psychol. Bull.* 40:385–422.

Herrnstein, R. J. 1970. On the Law of Effect. *J. Exp. Anal. Behav.* 13:243–266.

Kandel, E. R., and Gardner, D. 1972. The synaptic actions mediated by the different branches of a single neuron. In E. J. Kopin, ed., *Neurotransmitters*, vol. 50 of the Proceedings of the Association for Research in Nervous and Mental Diseases. Baltimore: Williams & Wilkins.

Kandel, E. R., and Spencer, W. A. 1968. Cellular neurophysiological approaches in the study of learning. *Physiol. Rev.* 48:65–134.

Kupfermann, I., Castellucci, V., Pinsker, H., and Kandel, E. 1970. Neural correlates of habituation and dishabituation of the gill-withdrawal reflex in *Aplysia. Science* 167:1743–1745.

Patterson, M. P., Cegavske, C. F., and Thompson, R. F. 1973. Effects of a classical conditioning paradigm on hind-limb flexor nerve response in immobilized spinal cats. *J. Comp. Physiol. Psychol.* 84:88–97.

Pinsker, H., Kupfermann, I., Castellucci, V., and Kandel, E. 1970. Habituation and dishabituation of the gill-withdrawal reflex in *Aplysia. Science* 167:1740–1742.

Prosser, C. L., and Hunter, W. S. 1936. The extinction of the startle responses and spinal reflexes in the white rat. *Am. J. Physiol.* 117:609–618.

Rescorla, R. A. 1967. Pavlovian conditioning and its proper control procedures. *Psychol. Rev.* 74:71–80.

Rexed, B. 1954. The cytoarchitectonic organization of the spinal cord in the cat. *J. Comp. Physiol.* 96:415–495.

Spencer, W. A., Thompson, R. F., and Neilson, D. R., Jr. 1966. Decrement of ventral root electrotonus and intra-cellularly recorded postsynaptic potentials produced by integrated cutaneous afferent volleys. *J. Neurophysiol.* 29:253–274.

Thompson, R. F., Groves, P. M., Teyler, T. J., and Roemer, R. A. 1973. A dual-process theory of habituation: theory and behavior. In H. V. S. Peeke and M. J. Herz, eds., *Habituation.* New York: Academic Press.

Thompson, R. F., and Spencer, W. A. 1966. Habituation: A model phenomenon for the study of neuronal substrates of behavior. *Psychol. Rev.* 73:16–43.

Wall, P. D. 1958. Excitability changes in afferent fiber terminations and their relation to slow potentials. *J. Physiol.* (London) 142:1–21.

Zucker, R. S. 1972. Crayfish escape behavior and central synapses. II. Physiological mechanisms underlying behavioral habituation. *J. Neurophysiol.* 35:621–737.

10

The Goldfish as a Model Experimental Animal for Studies of Biochemical Correlates of the Information-Storage Process

Victor E. Shashoua

Introduction

The nervous system has, as one of its major functions, the ability to reduce environmental information into a form that can be recorded and permanently stored. How is this accomplished? Are there any biochemical correlates of this function? If we assume that the process of information storage can ultimately lead to a modification of the nervous system, then it follows that the biochemical components of the system, which are the only ones available, must be used in some way to establish the change.

General Characteristics of Brain as a Tissue

Before we review the work carried out with the goldfish, it is important to point out a number of features of brain tissue that distinguish it from other tissues in an organism. First of all an outstanding characteristic is its anatomical complexity and organization. Unlike other organs such as liver or kidney, where a relatively few types of cells are arranged in a repetitive structure, the brain has the two general classes of cells (neurons and glia), with many subclasses. Each cell has many processes organized in a unique pattern of arborization for forming discrete interneuronal associations. The vast connective network linking these elements in various types of synaptic configurations leads us to ask whether each cell in the system should perhaps be regarded as a separate entity with its own unique pattern of connections.

Biochemically the brain is a dynamic organ. There is a constant turnover of its protein and RNA macromolecules. This occurs in spite of the fact that there is hardly any cell division in adult brain tissue. The

V. E. Shashoua, Biological Research Laboratory, McLean Hospital, Belmont, MA, 02178. Research for this paper was supported by the Grant Foundation and the National Institutes of Health NINDS.

average half-life of brain protein molecules is about fourteen days (Lajtha, 1964). Such a rapid rate of protein turnover requires an equally fast rate of RNA synthesis. It is estimated that the half-life of brain RNA is about three hours (Appel, 1967). In fact the only stable biochemical components in brain tissue are the DNA molecules, so that it is hard to rationalize how molecules other than DNA could be used in any mechanism for the permanent storage of information.

A most interesting aspect of brain metabolism becomes apparent when we consider the pattern in which the DNA in the genome is utilized. Investigations in a number of laboratories (Bondy and Roberts, 1969; Hahn and Laird, 1971) have suggested that, in spite of the low rate of proliferation of cells in nervous tissue, the rate of transcription of DNA into RNA for later use in protein synthesis is extremely high. In fact, if one could measure the amount of DNA being transcribed in an average cell at a given instant, one would find it to be about 2% of the total DNA; in brain tissue this type of measurement suggests that about 8% of the DNA is being so used. Does this represent the maximum commitment and utilization of the genetic-information content of the organism in the brain?

These features of brain metabolism clearly raise the question of how its biochemical metabolism can be responsive to environmental inputs. More specifically, is there a way in which the search for biochemical correlates of learning can be organized to take account of these features of brain metabolism? How can the acquisition of a new pattern of behavior influence a biochemical process? The following hypothetical model for the process of information storage was devised in order to explore these questions.

A Theoretical Model for Information Processing and Storage
A number of hypotheses have been proposed for the process of information storage in the brain. The early work of Flexner, Flexner, and Stellar (1963) suggested that there are two critical phases in the formation of a new memory. The first is "short-term memory," which is not sensitive to inhibitors of protein synthesis, and the second is "long-term memory," which is sensitive to inhibitors of protein synthesis such as puromycin and cycloheximide. Many studies of the time

sequence of delivery of the inhibitors relative to the time of training have been carried out (Flexner et al., 1964, 1968; Agranoff et al., 1966, 1967; Barondes et al., 1964, 1966; Cohen et al., 1966).

In an analysis of these studies the following hypothetical scheme was devised for the coupling of the information-storage process with brain metabolism (Shashoua, 1972). In this scheme (see Figure 10.1) environmental information, as detected by the heat, light, chemical, and mechanical sensory receptors of an organism, is converted by a series of four transduction steps into a long-term "metabolic demand signal" that is specific to the state of information recording in the particular neural circuits being used. This demand signal is postulated to act as a "trigger" that elicits, through two additional transduction steps, the synthesis of proteins for the modification of membranes in the nervous system. Each of the transduction steps outlined is a multicomponent and multistage event representing a phase in the continuous processing of the input into a suitable biochemical form for storage.

The basic assumption of the model is that the brain selects the *new* from the *old* features of the environment by using filters that allow only "novel" aspects of a given input to be transmitted to the next processing level. Thus distinct biochemical changes leading to cellular modifications occur only in the specific cells committed to new information. All other cells in the path of the input may increase their metabolic rate only in a manner characteristic of an increased "use" function. This model for information processing has been derived from the following considerations.

In the first stage information from the sensory receptors is transduced into a generalized type of output that is in an "electrical-time" mode, i.e., into the digital pulse output of neurons. The information-storage capacity in this mode is quite limited because the same receptor system that produces a given segment of information must be used over again in generating the next segment of a message. Thus the neuronal spike trains must be quickly converted into another mode of temporary information storage.

The most likely transduction process to occur at this stage is the conversion of the temporal coding pattern into a *spatial* array of electrical states. This is supported by findings that digital spike-train

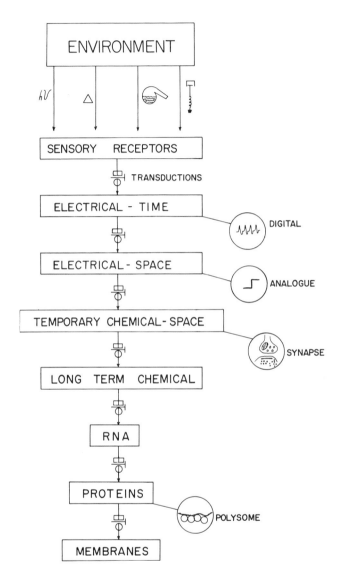

Figure 10.1 A diagram of the transduction processes in the nervous system. The symbols for environmental inputs represent light, heat, chemical, and mechanical inputs. Each transduction process characterizes a stage in the information-processing mechanism of the nervous system. These are considered to have specific time constants and to be the result of a multicomponent event representing the transit status of information.

inputs are converted to analogue signals (Grundfest, 1969; Werner and Mountcastle, 1965). Thus, at this stage the information is considered to be a distribution of "space charges" in a three-dimensional network involving many different brain areas. One fact that supports such a notion is the effect of electroconvulsive shock (ECS) in "erasing" short-term memory storage if applied within 10 sec after training in the rat (Chorover and Schiller, 1965). Additional experiments suggest that this susceptibility of the memory trace to disruption by ECS can last as long as 30 to 70 sec (Quartermain et al., 1965; McGaugh, 1966).

The third transduction process involves the conversion of the electrical-space state into a "chemical-space" state. By this means the electrical elements of the input generate a chemical signal at the same loci where the electrical charges were present. These temporary chemical changes may be at the synaptic sites, where a chemical coupling between pre- and postsynaptic sites can occur. There are many obvious candidates for such chemical changes, including changes in the concentration of transmitter substances or even in the production of small peptide molecules for signaling (Ungar, 1970). Temporary ionic changes would no doubt also be involved in the coupling.

A variety of time constants may define the lifetimes of the primary processes involved in encoding the chemical-space mode, and these time constants may depend on which indoleamines, catecholamines, or peptide hormones are used in the particular neural circuits involved in specifying the new input.

The fourth transduction process is the means by which events occurring at the cell membrane are communicated to the cell nucleus. Thus the temporary chemical-space mode is converted into a "long-term chemical" signal. At this stage the specific nature of the information encoded by a particular cell is essentially lost, and the function of the long-term chemical is simply to transmit to the cell nucleus a biochemical demand change for specific membrane proteins. Adenosine cyclic 3′,5′-monophosphate (cAMP) may have such a function in the nervous system (Shashoua, 1971). This function for cAMP is supported by a variety of findings indicating that electrical stimulation of the superior cervical ganglia (McAfee et al., 1971) or of brain-tissue slices

(Kakiuchi et al., 1969) can give rise to increased cAMP levels in nervous tissue. In addition brain-tissue slices can be stimulated to synthesize cAMP by catecholamines, particularly norepinephrine. As shown in Figure 10.1, the function of the long-term chemical is to signal the cell nucleus to synthesize RNA, which is to be used in subsequent steps for the synthesis of proteins needed to modify cell membranes in the last step of the information processing.

There are a number of molecules that could be considered for use as the long-term metabolic demand signal. Each molecule in this category might be specific to a class of neural circuits. Thus cAMP might be specific to norepinephrine and dopamine circuits (Shashoua, 1971), and is very likely specific to serotonin circuits as well. Recent studies (Kuo et al., 1972) suggest that guanosine cyclic 3',5'-monophosphate might be involved in acetylcholine circuits. And there might well be other types of metabolic demand signal, not necessarily nucleotides (Ungar, 1970), that are used in this type of function. From the experiments with cAMP the time constant for this stage appears to be about 2–3 hr since RNA synthesis shows a maximum change at about 3 hr following intracerebral administration of the drug, while there are no effects after 10 hr.

The transduction step from the long-term chemical signal to RNA synthesis has been reviewed by Glassman (1969). At this stage the integrity of the information is no longer preserved. The membrane structures, which in the third stage are involved in generating the chemical-space signal, are essentially withdrawn from receiving further inputs and function in a holding pattern until the metabolic systems can produce proteins to fix these patterns permanently. Thus the third stage may have one time constant governing the long-term chemical signal to the nucleus and another longer time constant during which the holding pattern awaits modification by proteins. Such a notion is supported by the findings of Deutsch (1971) that anticholinesterases have both short- and long-term effects.

The sixth stage is one in which mRNA is used for the synthesis of proteins. The time constant for this stage has been specified in a variety of experiments (Barondes et al., 1964; Agranoff et al., 1966) through the use of protein-synthesis inhibitors to prevent long-term memory storage.

Again a number of time constants can be deduced from experimental data, ranging from as little as 3 hr to about 10 hr (see Table 10.1). This may be dependent on the experimental animal used and the difficulty of the task to be remembered.

The last stage in the information processing is the assemblage of proteins into membrane elements at the chemical-space sites within the nervous system. The changes that may occur include a modification of the postsynaptic membranes and the production of more synaptic vesicles in a given neural circuit; they may also include the production of the new dendritic or axonal outgrowth and an increase in myelination of specific axons. In a recent paper by Roberts, Flexner, and Flexner (1970) it was shown that, when puromycin is administered 24 hr after a training session, the peptidyl derivative formed by the disruption of protein synthesis remains within the nervous tissue, causing amnesia for periods of as long as 30 days. Intracerebral saline injections during this period, however, can restore the memory, probably by releasing the puromycin peptides from their membrane-bound sites. Roberts, Flexner, and Flexner believe that these puromycin peptides have binding characteristics similar to norepinephrine. If, in fact, this occurs, then the puromycin peptides might interfere with the process of assembling membranes from newly synthesized proteins. This type of binding suggests that the time constant for the final transduction process can be quite long.

In this proposed mechanism information specificity is provided by the neural circuitry, while biochemical events define the means for their modification. Essentially the message writes itself, and the biochemical changes constitute a "repair" mechanism by which classes of proteins and their modifications are deposited at the same membrane sites, which are specified in the circuits depicting the new information. Thus message-specific proteins are not required. Moreover, once a structural change in a neural circuit has occurred, there is no necessity for long lifetimes for the proteins used. This is consistent with the relatively short half-life of 14 days reported by Lajtha (1964) for over 98% of brain proteins.

The proposed mechanism takes into account the dynamic nature of brain protein and RNA metabolism. Thus information recording in a

Table 10.1
Estimated time constants for the transduction processes

	1 EN to ET	2 ET to ES	3 ES to CS	4 CS to LC	5 LC to RNA	6 RNA to protein	7 Protein to membrane
Stimulated by				cAMP			
Inhibited by	ouabain (?)	ECS	anticholin-esterases		actinomycin D	puromycin cycloheximide	peptidyl puromycin
$\tau_{1/2}$ range		10–70 sec	min to hr	up to 2–3 hr	15 min to hr	3–10 hr	up to 30 days
References		Chorover et al. (1965) Quartermain et al. (1965) McGaugh (1966)	Deutsch (1971)	Shashoua (1971)	Hydén (1962) Glassman (1969) Agranoff (1967) Shashoua (1970)	Flexner et al. (1963) Barondes et al. (1966) Agranoff et al. (1966) Hydén (1968) Shashoua (1972)	Roberts et al. (1965)

Abbreviations: EN, environment; ET, electrical time; ES, electrical space; CS, chemical space; LC, long-term chemical; ECS, electroconvulsive shock; cAMP, cyclic adenosine monophosphate; $\tau_{1/2}$, half-life.

biochemical sense becomes a "microevent" in brain development. After a membrane change has occurred, its components become part of the overall structure of the brain and enter into the ongoing dynamics of brain metabolism, regenerating at the same general rate as other brain structures. In this way the specialized information-recording function of nervous tissue can utilize processes and substrates that may be common to all cells but are maximally developed in brain.

The Design of an Experimental Model System

There are three factors that must be considered in the selection of a model system for testing the foregoing hypothesis: (1) the experimental organism, (2) the type of behavioral task to be used for the training, and (3) the biochemical parameters to be used for the correlative studies.

If we hope to extrapolate our results to human memory, we must choose an experimental organism sufficiently high in the phylogenetic scale that memory is formed fairly rapidly and remains stable for weeks after the training experience. In our experiments the goldfish was selected because it combines good learning with a relative simplicity of brain anatomy. Goldfish have been widely used in studies of learning in both classical-conditioning (Behrend and Bitterman, 1964; Ingle, 1968) and operant-conditioning (Gonzalez and Bitterman, 1967) experiments. In addition there are a number of technical advantages to this choice: (1) Relatively large groups of animals can be used, so that behavioral or biochemical variations between individual animals can be averaged out experimentally. (2) Since adult goldfish can be small (7–8 g), a minimum quantity of radioactive label is required. (3) Labeling the brains of goldfish by direct intraventricular injection does not require major surgery. The anatomical features of the goldfish brain, such as the optic tectum, the cerebellum, and the vagal lobes, can be seen through the thin walled skull of the animal, and it is relatively easy to inject the label at a given site. (4) The goldfish brain is quite small (70 mg), so that a label, or any chemical for that matter, injected into the ventricle does not have to diffuse over large distances. (5) Drugs such as puromycin, actinomycin D, etc., which, at active doses, can be quite lethal or at least cause severe illness in mammals, can be used in goldfish without any observable effect on the ability of the animals to learn new tasks.

In order to promote the largest possible biochemical change the learning test should present a difficult challenge and maximally stimulate the nervous system of the animal. In our experiments this was achieved by using the float-training task (Shashoua, 1968). Here a foamed polystyrene float (a 0.7-cm cube) was sutured at the ventral surface of the experimental animals (7–8 g in weight) at a point 1 mm caudal to the first pair of lateral fins. Figure 10.2 illustrates the sequence of adaptation of the goldfish to the task. In stage I the animals are upside down. This is followed by a period of struggling during which the animals train to

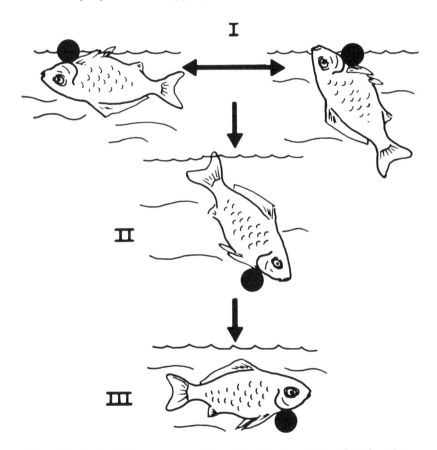

Figure 10.2 The float-training experiment for goldfish. Stage I corresponds to the naive state; the animals are upside down. Stage II is the 50% trained level; the animals swim constantly at a 45° angle. Stage III is the 100% trained level; the animals swim in a horizontal posture.

swim at a 45° angle in an upright position to achieve stage II of the task. This usually requires one hour and is followed by a varying time interval up to a total of four hours for the animals to assume stage III (horizontal swimming). This type of training obviously stimulates both vestibular and lateral line systems and presumably challenges those integrative centers, such as cerebellum, that participate in the coordination of new motor movements. The result of the training is a new behavioral pattern that produces a novel set of coordinated swimming movements.

As for the biochemical parameter to be used in a correlative study with the fish's new behavior, we decided to select first a general type of reaction characteristic of a wide variety of cells present in the nervous system. (This seemed preferable to a search for more specific molecules, limited to a relatively few cells in specific neural circuits, since these would be almost impossible to find even by the techniques of radioactive labeling.) One such parameter is the pattern of RNA synthesis. A number of investigators have suggested that there is a direct relationship between brain RNA and protein metabolism on the one hand and the mechanism by which new patterns of behavior are stored within neural tissue on the other (Hydén and Egyhazi, 1962; Shashoua, 1968). Indicative findings include: (1) an increase in RNA synthesis during learning (Bateson and Rose, 1972; Glassman, 1969); (2) the formation of RNA with a unique base composition during training (Hydén and Egyhazi, 1962; Shashoua, 1970b); and (3) a requirement for brain protein synthesis during the consolidation step of a new behavioral pattern (Flexner et al., 1963; Flexner and Flexner, 1968; Agranoff, 1967; Agranoff et al., 1965; Barondes and Cohen, 1964; Barondes and Jarvik, 1966; Cohen et al., 1966). However, it has not as yet been possible to distinguish changes occurring within the nervous system that reflect the assimilation of new information from changes that play only a supporting function. Thus the model system of choice must be adaptable to behavioral controls for such nonspecific factors as increased sensory stimulation, intense physical exercise, possible emotional stress, and the effect of performance on the biochemical changes observed.

Experimental Studies with the Goldfish

In our laboratory the goldfish experimental-model system was used to study biochemical correlates of the learning process. The float-training task was used as the behavioral experiment for an investigation of brain RNA changes during the acquisition of new swimming skills. This type of study focuses upon the transductional step, in our working model, in which long-term chemical changes are communicated to the cell nucleus to signal a change in the pattern of RNA synthesis. Thus the mechanism by which events occurring at cell membranes can generate a change in the biochemistry of brain tissue was explored.

In this kind of investigation it is important to distinguish changes that result in the synthesis of specific RNA molecules from those that produce general changes in the rate of RNA synthesis. Thus the effects of inducing other "behavioral states" that do not themselves represent learning must be dissociated from any results that are specifically due to the learning. It is well known that motor activity (Hydén, 1943), visual stimulation (Bok, 1970), electrical stimulation (Berry and Cohen, 1972), sleep (Vitale-Neugebauer et al., 1970), hibernation (Holmgren and Holmgren, 1968), and neuronal regeneration (Oderfield-Nowak and Niemierko, 1969; Haddad et al., 1969) can result in shifts of the amount of RNA synthesized, as measured by the amount of radioactive precursor incorporated into new RNA molecules (see Tables 10.2 and 10.3). In such experiments, however, there is no evidence to suggest that specific types of RNA molecules are produced. Thus a measure of the total quantity of RNA synthesized in a given situation is not a useful parameter for determining how learning influences RNA metabolism.

It is essential to design the experiments so as to obtain evidence for the synthesis of specific RNA macromolecules (Shashoua, 1970a). This can be accomplished by using the double-labeling technique. In this method (see Figure 10.3) groups of seven experimental animals are labeled intracerebrally with uridine-5 H^3 and an equal number of control animals are labeled with uridine-2 C^{14}. After the experimental group has been trained for seven hours, their brains are removed and homogenized with an equal number of control brains. The homogenates are fractioned into three components: nuclear, cytoplasmic, and synaptosomal (Shashoua, 1973). The RNA associated with each of these fractions is then isolated and purified (Shashoua, 1974a). The products are analyzed by ultracentrifugation to give sucrose-density-gradient patterns that separate the macromolecules according to their molecular weights. Figure 10.4 shows typical sucrose-density-gradient patterns and the

Table 10.2
General stimulation and RNA changes

	Animal	Label	Locus	RNA changes	Reference
Motor activity					
Running to exhaustion	guinea pig	none	spinal motor neurons	–	Hydén (1943)
Cyclic rotation	rat	none	Dieters-cell vestibular neurons	+ 5 to 20%	Hydén (1943)
Vestibular stimulation (constant rotation, 90 min)	goldfish	none	Mauthner-cell axon	–40%	Jakoubek and Edström (1965)
Constant swimming, 5 hr	barracuda	none	spinal motor neurons	+20%	Hydén (1964)
Constant swimming, 4 hr	goldfish	orotic acid	total brain	no base composition change	Shashoua (1971)
Visual stimuli					
Intense light	frog	cytidine	retinal rods	–50%	Bok (1970)
10 min exposure to light of dark-adapted animals	rat	uridine		+ 30 to 50% on large polysomes	Appel (1967)
Electrical stimulus					
3000 impulses through axonal inputs	*Aplysia*	uridine	R2-cell abdominal ganglia	+67%	Berry and Cohen (1972)

Table 10.3
Nonlearning behavioral and neurosurgical effects on RNA metabolism

	Animal	Label	Locus	RNA changes	References
Sleep	rabbit	orotic acid	cortex	+ in 28 to 50 S in polysome region in sleep	Vitale-Neugebauer et al. (1970)
Circadian rhythm	rat	none	brain, pineal, heart	RNA polymerase +44% at midnight	Merritt and Sulkowski (1970)
KCl-induced convulsions	goldfish	orotic acid	brain	no base composition change	Shashoua (1970)
Hibernation (cold-induced)	snail	none	neurons in visceral ganglion	−700%	Holmgren and Holmgren (1968)
Cold-induced epileptogenic foci	rabbit	uridine	cortex	− in neuronal nuclei; + in cytoplasm (autoradiographic analysis)	Engel and Morrell (1970)
Hypophysectomy	rat	uridine	brain stem and liver	decrease in high-molecular-weight RNA in polysomes	Gispen et al. (1970)
Axonal regeneration (after crush)	rat and cat	none	sciatic nerve	increase due to Schwann-cell proliferation	Oderfield-Nowak et al. (1969)
Neuronal regeneration (after axonal transection)	mouse	uridine	hypoglossal neuron	+75% after 3 days	Haddad et al. (1969)
Optic-nerve transection	chick	uridine	optic lobes	+ up to 17 days	Bondy and Margolis (1970)

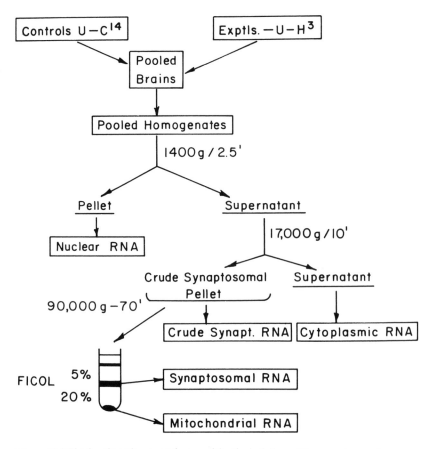

Figure 10.3 The fractionation procedure used for the isolation of the synaptosomal, nuclear, and cytoplasmic RNA components in a double-labeling type of experiment. The preparation is carried out at 0°C using 0.32 M sucrose as the homogenization medium. The RNA is isolated and purified from each fraction for use in ultracentrifugal analyses by sucrose-density-gradient sedimentation methods.

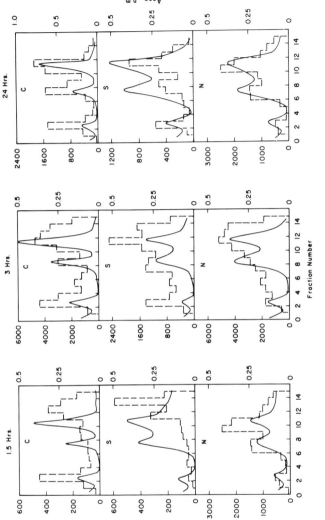

Figure 10.4 Sedimentation patterns of the cytoplasmic, synaptosomal, and nuclear RNA fractions obtained by ultracentrifugation in a 15 to 30% sucrose gradient for 18 hr at 0°C. The solid lines show the optical-density profiles (A_{260} nm) and the dashed lines depict the pattern of incorporation of uridine for the time points 1.5 hr, 3 hr, and 24 hr.

incorporation of labeled uridine into each of the nuclear, cytoplasmic, and synaptosomal fractions for the case of a single-label precursor. These data show the presence of transfer RNA together with two ribosomal RNA peaks in the gradients. The time course of synthesis of the RNA molecules illustrates the pattern of distribution and equilibration of the labeled products.

The double-labeling procedure for analysis of the pattern of RNA synthesis takes advantage of the fact that all processing variables are common to both experimental and control animals. The ratio of H^3 to C^{14} in each fraction of the gradient is independent of the composition of the metabolic pool since such changes merely raise the quantity of uridine in all RNA fractions and thus shift the ratio equally for all species of RNA. As shown in Figure 10.5, the ratio H^3/C^{14} is therefore constant for a control vs. control group of animals. The use of the double-labeling method, therefore, confines the biochemical investigation to changes in RNA molecules with a specific molecular weight.

Results from Double-Labeling Studies
In preliminary studies it was found that the most pronounced RNA changes occur in the synaptosomal and cytoplasmic RNA fractions. Figure 10.5 shows the results for a sucrose-density-gradient pattern of the RNA associated with the synaptosomal fraction. The lower part of the figure shows the distribution of RNA labeled with uridine C^{14} obtained from the experimental animals and that of the RNA labeled with uridine-5 H^3 from the controls. It is clear that there are two species of macromolecules that are present to a greater extent in the experimental group. The sedimentation properties of these molecules indicate that they are not ribosomal RNA. Plots for the ratio of labels in a control vs. control group (C/C) and an experimental group which did not learn the task vs. control, $(E/C)_{N.L.}$, give straight lines, indicating that no specific changes in the pattern of RNA synthesis occurred in these experiments.

Table 10.4 summarizes the types of results for the specific RNA changes obtained during learning. The data demonstrate that substantial RNA changes do occur during training, corresponding to an average increase of 47% at the specific RNA peaks. This becomes 4.8% in terms

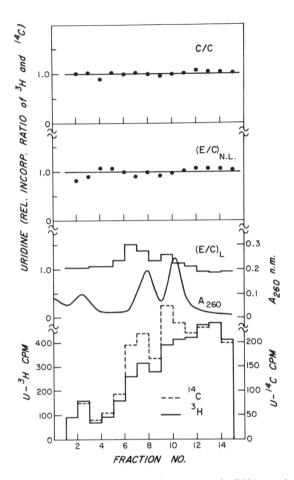

Figure 10.5 Sucrose-density-gradient patterns for RNA associated with the synaptosomal fraction. The optical-density pattern (A_{260}) shows the presence of tRNA and the ribosomal RNA peaks at 18s and 28s. The gradient was separated into fifteen fractions and the trichloroacetic-acid-precipitable RNA of each fraction was filtered on milipore filters and hydrolyzed with alkali; the quantity of H^3 and C^{14} label in each fraction was then determined by liquid-scintillation methods. The pattern of distribution of these isotopes is shown at the bottom of the figure. In two regions of the gradient an increase in uridine incorporation occurs for the experimental group. The relative ratios for the labels are displayed in the $(E/C)_L$ graph, where the 13s and 23s peaks show a 50% and 30% increase, respectively. The upper part of the figure shows the results for a control vs. control group (C/C). A constant ratio for the relative incorporation of H^3 and C^{14} into C/C indicates that there are no technical artifacts introduced in the procedure. This method of analysis also eliminates any variation due to pool changes since these would merely move the H^3/C^{14} ratio up or down throughout the gradient without producing any peaks. The figure also shows the results for a group of experimental goldfish (E) that did not learn the float-training task (i.e., $(E/C)_{N.L.}$); no relative change was observed here.

of the total RNA synthesized in the brain (i.e., the percent of total radioactive uridine incorporated). Clearly there is a specific RNA change for the experimental group of animals.

Control Experiments

The fact that a specific RNA change occurs in the experimental group of animals cannot be taken as evidence that this change is due to the learning. The float-training procedure is certainly stressful to the animals. In addition the goldfish work very hard during their attempts to learn the task. As a control for the "work" performed during the task, a study of the pattern of RNA synthesis was carried out for the goldfish that swam vigorously in a whirlpool for a period of 4–7 hr after injection

Table 10.4
Goldfish brain RNA changes during training

Experiment number[a]	Type[b]	RNA % at peak[c]	% of total[d]	Training score (%)	Remarks
1S	E/C	+ 65	1.6	55	learning
2S	E/C	+ 50	2.2	70	learning
3C	E/C	+ 45	7.0	50	learning
4C	E/C	+ 30	4.0	52	learning
5C	E/C	+ 60	6.5	58	learning
6C	E/C	+ 45	8.0	64	learning
7C	E/C	+ 35	4.0	55	learning
8–16	C/C				controls
17S	E/C			22	nonlearning
18S	E/C			25	nonlearning
19C	E/C			28	nonlearning
20C	E/C			80	pretrained control
21C	W/C				work control
22C	S/C				stress control

[a] Each experiment summarizes the data for the analyses of the sucrose gradients of the RNA from seven animals labeled with uridine-5 H^3 and seven animals labeled with uridine-2 C^{14}. (S = synaptosomal RNA; C = cytoplasmic RNA.)
[b] E/C, experimental vs. control groups; C/C, control vs. control groups; W/C, work vs. control groups; S/C, stressed vs. control groups. In each case the double-labeling method was used.
[c] The percent at peak represents the ratio of labels obtained for one fraction at the position of maximum RNA change. This occurred at two positions in the gradient (13S and 23S).
[d] This represents the fraction of the total incorporated label that is associated with peaks in the double-labeling experiments.

of the uridine (Shashoua, 1971). A double-labeling experiment of this type is reported in Table 10.4, experiment 21C. Here no specific RNA peaks were found, indicating that swimming to exhaustion in this situation does not produce the same type of result as the float-training situation. As a control for the effects of "stress" on brain RNA metabolism a variation of the training experiment was used in which the animals were sutured to a very large float (a 1.7-cm cube for the 7–8 g animals). In this situation the animals struggle unsuccessfully against the float but cannot achieve a horizontal swimming posture. The animals were also labeled for 7 hr using the double-labeling method. Under these stressful conditions no specific RNA changes were found (Table 10.4, experiment 22C).

In another control experiment we examined the pattern of RNA synthesis for animals performing a previously learned task. In this experiment the goldfish were first trained for a period of 48 hr without radioactive label; then after a two-day rest period they were labeled with the RNA precursors and retested with the regular floats. As shown in experiment 20C in Table 10.4, no specific RNA peaks were obtained. Thus mere performance of the float-compensation task, when new learning is not involved, does not produce the RNA changes.

Experiments 17S, 18S, and 19C in Table 10.4 reinforce this last point by providing data for animals that did not learn the standard float task. These groups received the label and float at the same times as those groups that learned the task, but their training scores did not change from their naive states by more than 15%. Such experiments seem to show that it is essential for the fish to master the challenge of the float before a specific RNA change can be detected.

The results show that the neural transduction process that results in the synthesis of a new RNA does produce *specific* RNA changes. We cannot, at the present stage of our knowledge, conclude that these changes are due exclusively to the learning component of the behavior. We can say, however, that certain types of behavioral experiment do not produce RNA changes. These include situations in which the animals do not learn, situations in which the animals are presented with a stressful but impossible task to solve, situations in which the animals perform a well-known task, and finally situations in which they merely swim vigorously. According to our theoretical view the specific RNA molecules synthesized may later be used for protein synthesis. In addition the fact that there are two specific RNA molecules formed suggests that there must be a minimum of two protein molecules involved in the consolidation process of new patterns of behavior.

References

Agranoff, B. W. 1967. Agents that block memory. In G. C. Quarton, T. Melnechuk, and F. O. Schmitt, eds., *The neurosciences—A study program.* New York: Rockefeller University Press.

Agranoff, B. W., Davis, R. E., and Brink, J. J. 1965. Memory fixation in the goldfish. *Proc. Natl. Acad. Sci. U.S.A.* 54:788.

Appel, S. H. 1967. Turnover of brain messenger RNA. *Nature* (London) 215:1253.

Barondes, S. H., and Cohen, H. D. 1966. Puromycin effect on successive phases of memory storage. *Science* 151:594.

Barondes, S. H., and Jarvik, M. E. 1964. The influence of actinomycin-D on brain RNA synthesis and on memory. *J. Neurochem.* 11:187.

Bateson, P. P. G., and Rose, S. P. R. 1972. Effects of early experience on regional incorporation of precursors into RNA and protein in the chick brain. *Brain Res.* 39:449.

Behrend, E. R., and Bitterman, M. E. 1964. Avoidance-conditioning in the fish: Further studies of the CS-US interval. *Am. J. Psychol.* 77:15.

Berry, R. W., and Cohen, M. J. 1972. Synaptic stimulation of RNA metabolism in the giant neuron of *Aplysia californica. J. Neurobiol.* 3:209.

Bok, D. 1970. The distribution and renewal of RNA in retinal rods. *Invest. Ophthalmol.* 9:516.

Bondy, S. C., and Margolis, F. L. 1970. Effect of unilateral enucleation on protein and ribonucleic acid metabolism of avian brain. *Exp. Neurol.* 27:344.

Bondy, S. C., and Roberts, S. 1969. Developmental and regional variations in ribonucleic acid synthesis on cerebral chromatin. *Biochem. J.* 115:341.

Chorover, S. L., and Schiller, P. H. 1965. Short-term retrograde amnesia in rats. *J. Comp. Physiol. Psychol.* 59:73.

Cohen, H. D., Ervin, F., and Barondes, S. H. 1966. Puromycin and cycloheximide: Different effects on hippocampal electrical activity. *Science* 154:1557.

Deutsch, J. A. 1971. The cholinergic synapse and the site of memory. *Science* 174:788.

Engel, J., Jr., and Morrell, F. 1970. Turnover of RNA in normal and secondarily epileptogenic rabbit cortex. *Exp. Neurol.* 26:221.

Flexner, J. B., Flexner, L. B., and Stellar, E. 1963. Memory and cerebral protein synthesis in mice as affected by graded amounts of puromycin. *Science* 141:57.

Flexner, L. B., and Flexner, J. B. 1968. Studies on memory: The long survival of peptidyl-puromycin in mouse brain. *Proc. Natl. Acad. Sci. U.S.A.* 60:923.

Gispen, W. H., de Wied, D., Schotman, P., and Jansy, H. S. 1970. Effects of hypophysectomy on RNA metabolism in rat brain stem. *J. Neurochem.* 17:751.

Glassman, E. 1969. The biochemistry of learning: An evaluation of the role of RNA and protein. *Annu. Rev. Biochem.* 38:605.

Gonzalez, R. G., and Bitterman, M. E. 1967. Asymptotic resistance to extinction in fish and rat as a function of interpolated retraining *J. Comp. Physiol. Psychol.* 63:342.

Grundfest, H. 1969. Synaptic and ephatic transmission. In G. H. Bourne, ed., *Structure and function of nervous tissue*, vol. 2. New York: Academic Press.

Haddad, A., Iucif, S., and Cruz, A. R. 1969. Synthesis of RNA in neurons of the hypoglossal nerve nucleus, after section of the axon, in mice. *J. Neurochem.* 16:865.

Hahn, W. E., and Laird, C. D. 1971. Transcription of nonrepeated DNA in mouse brain. *Science* 173:158.

Holmgren, R. U., and Holmgren, B. 1968. Relative RNA changes in snail macroneurons during experimental hibernation. *Brain Res.* 8:220.

Hydén, H. V. 1943. Protein metabolism in the nerve cell during growth and function. *Acta Physiol. Scand. [Suppl.]* 17:1.

Hydén, H. V. 1964. Biochemical and functional interplay between neuron and glia. In J. Wertis, ed., *Recent advances in biological psychiatry*, vol. 6. New York: Plenum.

Hydén, H. V., and Egyhazi, E. 1962. Nuclear RNA changes of nerve cells during a learning experiment in rats. *Proc. Natl. Acad. Sci. U.S.A.* 48:1366.

Hydén, H. V., and Egyhazi, E. 1968. The effect of tranylcypromine on synthesis of macromolecules and enzyme activities in neurons and glia. *Neurology* 18:732.

Ingle, D. 1968. Interocular integration of visual learning by goldfish. *Brain Behav. Evol.* 1:58.

Jacoubek, B., and Edstrom, J. E. 1965. RNA changes in the Mauthner axon and myelin sheath after increased functional activity. *J. Neurochem.* 12:845.

Kakiuchi, S., Rall, T. W., and McIlwain, H. 1969. The effect of electrical stimulation upon the accumulation of adenosine 3′, 5′-monophosphate in isolated cerebral tissue. *J. Neurochem.* 16:485.

Kuo, J.-F., Lee, T.-P., Reyes, P. L., Walton, K. G., Donnelly, T. E., Jr., and Greengard, P. 1972. Cyclic nucleotide-dependent protein kinases. *J. Biol. Chem.* 247:16.

Lajtha, A. 1964. Protein metabolism of the nervous system. *Int. Rev. Neurobiol.* 6:1.

McAfee, D. A., Schorderet, M., and Greengard, P. 1971. Adenosine 3′, 5′-monophosphate in nervous tissue: Increase associated with synaptic transmission. *Science* 171:1156.

McGaugh, J. L. 1966. Time-dependent processes in memory storage. *Science* 153:1351.

Merritt, J. H., and Sulkowski, T. S. 1970. Rhythmicity of RNA polymerase activity and RNA levels in nuclei of rat cerebral cortex. *J. Neurochem.* 17:1327.

Oderfeld-Nowak, B., and Niemierko, S. 1969. Synthesis of nucleic acids in Schwann cells as the early cellular response to nerve injury. *J. Neurochem.* 16:235.

Quartermain, D., Paolino, R. M., and Miller, N. E. 1965. A brief temporal gradient of retrograde amnesia independent of situational change. *Science* 149:1116.

Roberts, R. B., Flexner, J. B., and Flexner, L. B. 1970. Some evidence for the involvement of adrenergic sites in the memory trace. *Proc. Natl. Acad. Sci. U.S.A.* 66:310.

Shashoua, V. E. 1968. RNA changes in goldfish brain during learning. *Nature* (London) 217:238.

Shashoua, V. E. 1970a. Pattern of brain RNA synthesis during learning. *J. Cell Biol.* 47:188a.

Shashoua, V. E. 1970b. RNA metabolism in goldfish brain during acquisition of new behavioral patterns. *Proc. Natl. Acad. Sci. U.S.A.* 65:160.

Shashoua, V. E. 1971. Dibutyryl adenosine 3′, 5′-monophosphate effects on goldfish behavior and brain RNA metabolism. *Proc. Natl. Acad. Sci. U.S.A.* 68:2835.

Shashoua, V. E. 1972. Multistage transduction model for information processing in the nervous system. *Int. J. Neurosci.* 3:299.

Shashoua, V. E. 1973. The pattern of synthesis and distribution of membrane-bound RNA in brain synaptosomes. *Exp. Brain Res.* 17:139.

Shashoua, V. E. 1974a. Increased synthesis of specific RNA molecules in goldfish brain during training. *Brain Res.* (in press).

Shashoua, V. E. 1974b. RNA metabolism in brain. *Int. Rev. Neurobiol.* 16:183.

Ungar, G., ed. 1970. *Molecular mechanisms in memory and learning.* New York: Plenum.

Vitale-Neugebauer, A., Guiditta, A., Vitale, B., and Guinquinto, S. 1970. Pattern of RNA synthesis in rabbit cortex during sleep. *J. Neurochem.* 17:1263.

Werner, G., and Mountcastle, V. B. 1965. Neural activity in mechanoreceptive cutaneous afferents: Stimulus-response relations, Weber function, and information transmission. *J. Neurophysiol.* 28:359.

Index